D0853271

41–Love

ALSO BY SCARLETT THOMAS

FICTION

Our Tragic Universe
The End of Mr. Y
PopCo
Going Out
Bright Young Things
The Seed Collectors
Oligarchy

NONFICTION

Monkeys with Typewriters

41–LOVE

On Addictions, Tennis, and Refusing to Grow Up

Scarlett Thomas

COUNTERPOINT
Berkeley, California

41–Love

Copyright © 2021 by Scarlett Thomas
First hardcover edition: 2021

All rights reserved under International and Pan-American Copyright
Conventions. No part of this book may be used or reproduced in any manner
whatsoever without written permission from the publisher, except in the case of
brief quotations embodied in critical articles and reviews.

Library of Congress Cataloging-in-Publication Data
Names: Thomas, Scarlett, author.
Title: 41–love : on addictions, tennis, and refusing to grow up / Scarlett Thomas.
Other titles: Forty-one-love
Description: First hardcover edition. | Berkeley, California :
Counterpoint Press, 2021.
Identifiers: LCCN 2020053219 | ISBN 9781640094765 (hardcover) |
ISBN 9781640094772 (ebook)
Subjects: LCSH: Thomas, Scarlett. | Novelists, English—
21st century—Biography.
Classification: LCC PR6120.H66 Z46 2021 | DDC 823/.92 [B]—dc23
LC record available at https://lccn.loc.gov/2020053219

Jacket design by Kelly Winton
Book design by Jordan Koluch

COUNTERPOINT
2560 Ninth Street, Suite 318
Berkeley, CA 94710
www.counterpointpress.com

Printed in the United States of America

1 3 5 7 9 10 8 6 4 2

For Rod, with love

Though we would never wish the poisonous red shoes and the subsequent decrease of life onto ourselves or others, there is in its fiery and destructive center a something that fuses fierceness to wisdom in the woman who has danced the cursed dance, who has lost herself and her creative life, who has driven herself to hell in a cheap (or expensive) handbasket, and yet who has somehow held on to a word, a thought, an idea until she could escape her demon through a crack in time and live to tell about it.

—CLARISSA PINKOLA ESTÉS

CONTENTS

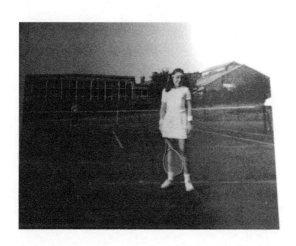

41–Love

Prologue

You can only start at the beginning if you know what the beginning is, but maybe this will do. It's a Wednesday in July 2013. I've arrived at the Indoor Tennis Centre for a tennis lesson. I last had a tennis lesson when I was fourteen, far away in the sweltering heat of Mexico, not long before I gave up playing seriously forever. I have just turned forty-one. I am wearing blue cotton Adidas shorts and a striped cotton tank top I hope doesn't make me look fat. I won't wear cotton for very long in this story—indeed, I will have to move on to "performance" fabrics quite soon—but it is how I begin. I have an old tennis racquet that cost about £25 from a funny little shop in Canterbury. The coach is a large, cheerful guy who is bouncing around teaching some kid, with brightly colored hoops and targets everywhere. He is running so late I almost say something—almost, but not quite. I am trying not to feel intimidated. This place is huge. Serious. Professional. Everything's green and smells of rubber or acrylic. There is a bulletin board with team lists printed on it. Ladies 1. Mixed 1. Ladies 2. *Imagine* . . . But I don't let myself. Not yet.

My turn, at last. I have no idea how much is wrong with the way I hit the ball. My whole technique is modeled on the way the cool older guys used to play at the local hard courts in Chelmsford when I was a kid. Flat, low, skimming the net. Nowadays everyone plays the ball earlier, harder, with topspin. But I don't yet know any of this. I am just pleased that I can hit the ball at all, that I can keep a rally going with this coach.

I stand a long way behind the baseline, waiting for the ball to come to me. It flies through the air (spinning over and over itself, although I cannot yet read spin), then bounces: beautiful, poetic, mathematical, as if all the laws of the universe were distilled into this one simple movement. It hits the ground, arcs, peaks, and then begins to drop. It's at the very last moment that I hit it, trying to remember what I learned all those years ago about "following through." I'm fast around the court, and I get to every ball, but I don't yet realize that this coach, Dan, is playing easy for me, playing down to me, because at this moment for him I am some random woman who has come along to maybe improve her game enough to be allowed to play with her husband, or her slightly better friend, or to join some social tennis club.

Of course my ambitions are greater than this, my ambitions that will soon build and eventually collapse like a vast, terrifying avalanche. At this moment, though, I just want to impress him. Embarrassingly, bizarrely, I want him to declare that he's never seen anyone so talented in all his years of coaching and . . . I don't know. Ask me to come back? Ask me to train for one of the teams? Just to praise one of my shots would be a start.

On the next court a younger, thinner blond coach is feeding

balls from a basket to a dark-haired woman who keeps laughing and missing her shots. *I am better than her,* I think. *I am not the worst person in here.* Their session ends before ours, and the blond guy grins and apologizes as he walks behind me with his basket of balls and his beaten-up old Dunlop racquet with the leather grip that I will later learn makes his fingers bleed when he plays in tournaments. The woman follows him, still laughing. Dan calls to her, something like, "How did you get on?" and she says, "Oh, I beat him again and he just can't handle it." It's pretty clear that he has let her win. Is this what coaches do with ladies who have £25 to spare for a lesson with them? Immediately, a yearning begins in me. One day I'm going to beat one of these coaches for real. I want to face one of these guys as their equal. I want them to *want* to hit with me.

A year or so later, when I am training for Seniors' Wimbledon, hitting with Dan as a friend, as his mixed doubles partner, he will look at me and say, "Did you have any idea, on that first day you came in here, that first session you had with me? Did you even *think* that you'd be here, that you'd have achieved all of this?" Of course I did—sort of—but I won't say that. By then I'll be thinking that whatever I achieve isn't good enough, and I'll be wracked with doubts and terrors and problems with my forehand, with my desperate need to win.

As I leave after that first session with my cheap racquet in my cheap bag, walking up the stairs feeling happy and complete in some way I haven't experienced for a long time, aching to play again as soon as possible but with various muscles beginning to go into spasm, I realize that someone's running up the stairs behind me. It's the blond guy. The other coach.

"You were hitting the ball nicely down there," he says.

"Thanks," I say. And then: "I'm Scarlett, by the way."

"Josh," he says. "See you again soon, I hope."

He passes me, and carries on running to wherever he's going.

1

The Indoor Tennis Centre

It is December 21, 2013. I am forty-one years old and I am just about to play in my first tennis competition. I've been half-joking, or maybe let's say three-quarters-joking, for the last few weeks that I am going to win this, the Indoor Tennis Centre Christmas Tournament Ladies' Singles. I have read books (always the first thing I do), weight-trained, studied strategy, watched tennis matches on YouTube. Initially, maybe back in November, I told myself, and my partner Rod, that I was going to win. But I didn't completely believe it, and as the thing approached I realized I was mad to think of victory, especially as one of the entrants—the favorite, in fact—was a teenage tennis star with a coach, supportive parents, and a string of victories behind her. When I looked at the list of entrants with my coach, Dan, he simply shook his head and said, "You'll have trouble beating her."

I've been playing tennis again for almost six months and I don't understand why I am not better. I mean, I'm good. I know that. Inside my head I'm really, really good, but my inner picture has not yet translated to actual results. I've played a couple of disastrous league matches by now and become a regular at Dan's Monday-night "Recreational Session." These would be called club nights, except the

Indoor Tennis Centre isn't a club, as such: it's a pay-and-play, council-run center that you can't join, exactly, but it does have teams. The Reccy sessions are clique-y and weird and I occasionally cry when I come home after them. Hayley, Dan's mixed doubles partner, is clearly his favorite. She hits the ball hard, and she knows how to do topspin. Then there's a bunch of large, confident women who hit the ball extremely hard and occasionally do drive volleys. And on the next court Becky Carter has her weekly coaching session with Josh.

The first time I saw Becky Carter I almost passed out with jealousy. She walked into the tennis center with a racquet handle sticking out of her backpack and everything, *everything*, from the angle of the racquet handle, to her sexy-naïve smile, to her blonde hair done up in a scruffy ponytail, was so perfect I wanted to die. Everyone was so pleased to see her. She'd been out with some kind of injury and this was her first session back. She was wearing little shorts with a tight top that showed her flat, muscular stomach. When she started hitting the ball with Josh it was like some flying martial arts film. She almost seemed like his equal. I wanted to do what she was doing so much that my brain couldn't understand that I wasn't in fact doing it. Of course, she has not entered the Christmas Tournament. Why would she?

My first match in the Christmas Tournament is against Karen, who has, she tells me, just been to do her family's weekly shop in Sainsbury's. To prepare for today, I have spent the previous day in a spa, had a full-body massage and a steam bath, drunk only two small glasses of red wine in the evening—although admittedly while sitting on a very hard chair for a long evening of performances based on Dickens at the local theatre—eaten two eggs for breakfast along with my usual "primal cereal," and done some visualization and, OK, a little bit of praying to the universe. I meant to meditate, but didn't. I have, however, watched a lot of videos of Federer on You-Tube. I love his backhand. It's one-handed, like mine. I have read and reread *The Inner Game of Tennis*, probably my favorite tennis book. It tells you to let go, relax, breathe, and let the mysterious inner part of you it calls "Self 2" play the game while you distract your ego by trying to read the writing on the tennis ball as it comes over the net toward you.

My initial mistake is in thinking that the fact that I have done all this and Karen has been to Sainsbury's means that I will win easily. I'm much more worried about Amie Tonkiss, the teenage tennis queen. But to be honest, I'm nervous as hell about the whole thing. I haven't really thought through my strategy, but if I had to put it into words, it would be something like "Keep getting the ball back and wait for your opponent to make a mistake." This is not the strategy I plan to take through my year of tennis (and at this moment I don't yet know I am going to have a year of tennis, nor that this is going to take me to the very brink of existence and sanity), but it is my strategy, sort of, for the Indoor Tennis Centre Christmas Tournament 2013. The only problem is that this is clearly also Karen's strategy. And she is just as patient and accurate as I am.

Another problem is that being careful and accurate is not much fun. There's no pace on the ball as it just plomps over the net and plomps back. I hit the ball so much harder in practice, with my male coach. I know that inside I have a game that is more aggressive, in which I hit harder, deeper, ground strokes that will force a shorter ball, which I can use to approach the net. But when I half-heartedly try this, my approach shot is weak. Karen, a good doubles player, just lobs me.

Those two glasses of wine the night before have made me dehydrated. It's too early for me. I don't usually play tennis at 10:00 a.m.

I like playing at approximately 3:00 p.m., which is when I have my weekly session with Dan Brewer, head coach at the Indoor Tennis Centre. I hit long and hard with him, but for some reason these rallies are leaving me gasping not just for water but for air. I've had way too much breakfast. The energy bars I brought with me are like 90 percent nuts. I can't digest nuts in this situation! After one long tiring point, I think I am going to throw up. I bend down to pretend to tie my shoelace just to give myself a moment to breathe. I am tanking. I am, possibly, dying. I have the beginnings of a blister that means I won't be able to walk tomorrow.

Karen wins the first three games. This is it. I am fucked.

My partner Rod is sitting at a green plastic table just beyond the tramlines, watching me play tennis for the first time ever. He is literally on the edge of his seat, although this isn't a very close match so far. He said that watching me play tennis would make him feel a bit like he does watching New Zealand's All Blacks, which is good. The other sport he gets very emotionally involved in is cricket, and at this point I'd rather be the New Zealand rugby team than its cricket team. But the All Blacks always win, or at least they have all the way through 2013, and here I am in what so far feels more like New Zealand's historic cricketing defeat in 1955, when they were bowled out for 26 (and which traumatized Rod for life). But what can I do? Karen is just playing very steadily. The rallies are punishing and they are long. I'm getting the ball back, I'm keeping it in, but it isn't working. I know I am better than this. Vague memories from childhood come wafting back. Was I always like this? Was I always better in practice than in matches and was that one of the reasons why . . . ?

After the third game changeover, I remind myself to do some basic things. Hit deeper, and more often to her backhand. Serve deep, too. Stay on my toes. I am still effectively a beginner and do not know even half the strategy I will know by the end of January, let alone what I will know by the end of next year. I have no second serve. No two-handed backhand. (I think my one-hander is pretty awesome, but the score-line begs to differ. Later in the year, Josh, my new coach, will just laugh at it.) But despite the better-in-practice thing, I do have a sort of history of winning singles matches. After all, I do have a natural ability for this beautiful game that I turned my back on so long ago, when I was fourteen and far from home, on a boarding school tennis court with Madonna hair and the wrong accent. I can see patterns in things. I "just know" where to hit the ball. I have recently beaten the local hard-hitter and queen-of-the-frightening-volley 6–2 in a practice game in which I definitely thought I'd be crushed. I thrashed a steady male club player 6–1. So why am I losing to someone who has just been round Sainsbury's?

I don't know how, but I take the next game. And the next one. Sometimes it's just about deciding that you really want *this* thing rather than some other thing. *I am going to win this tennis tournament*, I tell the universe. And if I am going to win the tournament, I need to win this set, this game, this point. The universe sighs and I draw level, but then Karen wins the next game, taking her to 4–3. I take the next game, and the next one. It's 5–4. I'm serving for the match, but I can't do it. We're level again at 5–5, and then again at 6–6. I had thought that if I could stay in it this long I would have some sort of advantage, given that I am more likely to be found in the gym than Sainsbury's. Most people find even a few games of singles tough, let alone twelve very long games with multiple deuces. But no, Karen looks as fresh as when we began, while I still feel a bit vomit-y. I can't remember the rules for a tiebreaker and neither can Karen but when we ask the organizer,

Margaret, she reminds us that there are no tiebreakers in this tournament. Someone simply has to go two games clear.

Because this isn't an official LTA (Lawn Tennis Association, Great Britain's governing body for tennis) tournament, just a bit of fun (albeit with big shiny trophies), the changeovers are pretty relaxed. I go over to Rod. Still on the edge of his seat, he tells me to please finish it off. Can I perhaps hit the ball harder? Target her backhand? Hit more outright winners rather than waiting for her to make a mistake? Karen and I have now been playing for almost two hours. We have quite a big audience, which is usually good for me—I like to perform—except one of them is an old woman with a blanket over her knees who has a particularly loud cackle that has been putting me off. As I guzzle the horrible orange juice and water mixture recommended by my personal trainer, people say things about how long the game is and generally praise my grit and stamina.

"I don't know how you're doing it," says someone.

"I think I'd die if it was me," says someone else.

But I am used to long, drawn-out things. I have just finished writing a novel, my ninth. I'm on sabbatical from the university job that recently seemed to be tipping me into alcoholism and mild obesity, and for the last few weeks my routine has been to write in the morning and then play tennis in the afternoon or the evening. It's like the perfect life. I have my weekly coaching session with Dan on Thursdays. I try to use the ball machine one day a week and then lift weights once or twice. I do have some grit and stamina. But do I have enough?

Back on court I lose a match point. I save a match point. Suddenly there are match points all over the place. We must be around 8–8 when one of my balls kisses the line and Karen calls it out. I'm pissed off but I know she is honest and nice, and if she saw it out, then she saw it out. Whatever. But it's unfortunate because it takes the score to 30–40. Break point. But as I go back to serve, she calls to me. Perhaps it was in, she says. Now she thinks about it, she realizes she called wrong. On such an important point you have to be sure, right? Her honesty saves me. From there I go on to win 10–8.

I am exhausted but there is still a lot of tournament left to play, especially as I'm down to play mixed doubles as well as singles. People are buying sausages and chips from the café in the leisure center upstairs and bringing them down on shiny white paper plates. Tim, my doubles partner, buys me tea in a Styrofoam cup, which has to be my changeover drink in the next match, which I realize is starting immediately. But I know that I can't win at doubles as well as singles. Since I came back to tennis in July, I have had the same two annoying injuries: knees and lower back, the same injuries all recreational tennis players seem to get. Neither has been too bad lately, but I have to pace myself. One of my calves is starting to cramp a little bit. I am the stronger player in what we jokingly refer to as the "Dream Team" but I can't give myself to this. Tim suffers badly from match nerves, knocking balls into the net that he would kill in practice. We lose our first match but at least my tea is nice.

My next singles opponent is Netball Hannah. She has just been bagelled (lost 6–0) by Amie Tonkiss and she isn't happy.

"I'm just so sick of being beaten," she's saying to Margaret and Dan. "I feel like such a bloody loser. I might just go home, to be honest. Why does everyone have to take it so seriously?" She looks at me. "It's just a bit of fun, right?"

"Er, yeah."

After I beat her 6–0, she does go home. Do I feel bad? Sort of. I've played my worst, slowest, most drippy tennis against her, which does make me feel pretty awful. I also have this strange new hunger in me: I would have felt like a loser had I dropped even one game to her. I am also convinced by the argument in *The Inner Game of Tennis* that you should go out and play your best every time, regardless of your opponent's level of skill or expectations. I suppose there'd be the odd exception. Perhaps playing a child. Although when I was a child I played tennis against my stepfather, Couze, and he beat me 6–0 most of the time. Every point I won against him meant something. If I took a game to deuce, it was a big achievement. My biggest problem at that age was that I couldn't bear the embarrassment of beating my friends, or random girls with names like Julie or Tracey, so I used to deliberately let them have points here, games there, until it was a more respectable 6–4. Although often this would go wrong and I would underestimate their actual ability and they would beat me.

A colleague of mine, feminist theorist Jan Montefiore, once told me about playing table tennis with one of her sons. "It was extraordinary," she said. "I was winning by nineteen points and then he came back to beat me 21–19." I remember thinking at the time how sweet this was, that she didn't know what had really happened, but as I write it now I realize that of course she must have known. People always know when they are being controlled and manipulated, even if it is meant in kindness. I hate it when Dan plays down to me in our coaching sessions. It's so unsatisfying. You never know if you have won a point on your own merit or because someone has taken pity on you. Luckily, Dan doesn't do it very often. Indeed, he bagelled me a couple of days before this tournament, to teach me something—probably humility. I point this out to Hannah before she leaves. There's no shame in it; it happens to us all.

"Yeah, well, just make sure you beat *her*," she says, nodding at Amie Tonkiss.

Someone tells me that Hannah barely took a point off Amie.

But next I have to play Kofo. She hits the ball hard—much harder than anyone I've played so far—but she makes a lot of errors. Still, she rushes the net a few times, and so do I, and there are lobs and volleys and passing shots and a bit of cheering from the audience, which is nice. It feels as if she is winning more points than she is, but in the end I beat her 6–1 in something of a blur. Rod has gone home long ago, unable to take the cold of the tennis center for the whole day, but now I text him to tell him that I am playing in the equivalent of a final. Although it's a round robin tournament, Amie and I are both unbeaten so far, so this will be the decider. In fact, if I win this—I won't, but if I do—I will have beaten everyone.

Rod and I only live around the corner from the ITC, and so he arrives, breathless and excited, about four minutes later. The match that follows is somehow more of a blur than the last one. Amie blitzes me in the first game and I know my winning run is about to come to an end. I relax at that point—and then I win my serve. She wins her next one and I win mine. We are level, which is a surprise. And then, suddenly, I break her serve. The type of steady tennis that I will spend the next year trying to stop playing works against Amie. I return the balls and she tries to hit winners. Sometimes they work, but more often they don't. I suspect she's having an off day but, extraordinarily, I am beating her quite easily. Rod shifts in his plastic chair. He looks more like he is watching rugby than cricket, even quietly cheering from time to time.

I win, 6–2.

So I have won the ladies' singles. I can't believe how happy I feel. It's definitely as good as publishing my first novel. Way better than my first kiss. I still have some doubles to play—against Amie and her father, which they win easily, and against Lee and the old lady with the blanket, which we do manage to win. Rod goes home to put a half bottle of champagne in the freezer. We will drink a further bottle of red in the local French restaurant afterward. When I tell him what it was like being given my trophy, he gets tears in his eyes and so do I.

It goes on the mantelpiece, right in the middle, and as I look at it there, I realize that at this moment, even with my new novel finished and my next promotion—the one that will make me a professor—almost due at the university, all I really want is another tennis trophy.

This is what is going to almost kill me.

•

The day after the Christmas Tournament I am in London for my new literary agency's party. One of my best friends, the novelist David Flusfeder, has like me recently defected to this agency. We meet in a pub beforehand and I tell him about my win, and what it means to me. He's not that sporty, but he gets it. After a couple of glasses of wine, he asks me whether I would rather win the Nobel Prize for Literature or score the winning goal in the FA Cup.

"You first," I say.

"But there's no question for me," he says.

"What, the Nobel?"

"No," he says, "the goal. I'd much rather score the goal."

He doesn't even play football, as far as I know. He's more likely to be found in a casino in Las Vegas taking part in a poker championship.

"I don't play football," I say. "I'm not sure I even like it."

"What about winning Wimbledon then?" he says.

Oh God. What indeed? What about that? Well, still the Nobel, right?

But when I ask people over the next few days and weeks, everyone—great feminists, choristers, academics, editors—chooses the FA Cup goal. A couple of them, Rod included, have to have it upgraded to the winning goal in the World Cup, but still choose the goal. But everyone in my family chooses the Nobel.

•

It is 12:45 p.m. on January 11, 2014. The match begins at 1:00 p.m. I am standing on Court 4 in the cold, hard, green emptiness of the Indoor Tennis Centre, entirely alone. I am wearing Stella McCartney for Adidas. I have painted my fingernails dark pink to artfully clash with my bright red shoes. I have taped my probably infected toe and put Band-Aids on the worst pressure points on each foot. My black Adidas bag is packed with knee braces, spare sweatbands, electrolyte pills, magnesium spray, arnica gel, more Band-Aids, chocolate, water, and more ibuprofen than you could safely ingest in a week. I have been warming up in the gym for the last half hour, listening to uplifting music, or my idea of uplifting music: mainly The The and clubby, drug-reference-heavy stuff from the early 1990s. I spent yesterday icing various parts of myself while reading a book called *Think to Win*. I have meditated, stretched, visualized. Sort of. I am ready to play tennis.

12:55. Still no one. I check my phone to see if someone has texted me to say the match has been canceled, but I'm pretty sure it has not. I arrange our two courts carefully. Eight plastic chairs altogether: two on either side of both ends of the net, with spaces left in the middle for where the umpires would go, if there were umpires. Once I finish scraping chairs around, the only sound left in the tennis center is from the kids in the park outside throwing rocks at the fire doors. At 12:59 there are faint sounds from the stairwell. It's the away team, arrived from somewhere near Rochester. At least, I assume they are the away team. I have never seen any of them before. But I don't really know who is playing on our team. They could even *be* our team, except there are four of them. I mumble things about water and toilets until our captain, Fiona, turns up. She has two tins of Head Championship balls pressed into her chest and a bag full of cakes and baguettes dangling from her wrist. She is also holding a piece of paper.

"I've got the match balls," she says. "But this is the wrong form, apparently, and I don't know how to fill it in."

"This is the away team," I say.

"Oh, hello," she says. "Long journey?"

One of my favorite tennis books at this moment is *Winning Ugly* by Brad Gilbert. I just got it for Christmas and devoured it on my parents' sofa between bottles of Vacqueyras wine and hot, frenzied games of table tennis. I read it on the train back, still drunk on my recent success, ready to slurp up anything, *anything* to do with tennis, my new love, my passion, my life. It was so good that when I got home, I read it again. I made notes. It explains in detail how to approach a competitive tennis match. It tells you what to pack in your bag, how to warm up, and why you should never serve first. It explains how many tennis racquets you should bring to a match and how they should be strung. It also cautions strongly against chatting with your opponents until after the match, but by the time we begin, everyone has looked at pictures of French Florence's puppy and the away team have started eating the baguettes that are supposed to be for afternoon tea. I was put in charge of cheese and biscuits, and these are sensibly stashed in the fridge in the café upstairs. One of our team has some pâté and cold meats at the bottom of her sports bag. It is impossible to tell how long they have been there.

I also have a book on doubles strategy, which is fascinating, although almost entirely irrelevant when playing with someone you have never met, let alone practiced with. Is it weird of me to think that the normal thing for a team to do in this situation would be to turn up half an hour early, decide who is playing with whom, warm up, get a bit of team spirit going, rock the home advantage? If it were up to me, each doubles pair would not just have played together before but would have trained together, probably going halves on a few coaching sessions involving traffic cones and diagrams. If it were up to me, my partner and I would be playing the Australian formation. We would fist-bump after every point. We would wear matching outfits, perhaps with tiaras. OK, not tiaras, but we might have a theme song. And we would certainly have a mantra. The person at the baseline would call soft but clever instructions to the person at the net . . .

"Does anyone have a spare tennis racquet?" asks Fiona. "I've left mine at home."

I have a spare tennis racquet. Of course I do. Brad Gilbert says you should always have a good spare (rather than your crappy ex-racquet) in case a string breaks during a match. This means I have two black Wilson 104 Blades, each strung at 55 lbs. (I have no idea what this means, but it looked good on the website.) Am I going to lend one of these racquets, my beautiful prized possessions, to Fiona? No, of course not. I am never going to let anyone touch these racquets apart from me. Venus and Serena use Blades. I bet they don't lend their racquets to other people. Or maybe they do. Maybe when you go through forty-one restrings in two weeks, as Serena did in Wimbledon 2013, or crack open a newly strung racquet whenever there are new balls, as most pro players do, you feel differently about them.

Did I ever kid myself at the beginning of all this, when I bought myself a tennis coaching session for my birthday last summer, that I wanted to play "social" tennis? I think so. I think I told myself that tennis would be a good way to meet new people in this strange seaside town in which I have felt cold, exposed, and isolated, sometimes to the point of tears. But I'd forgotten how competitive I am, and how much I want to win. And I know that this is my last chance to do the thing I love, the thing that I was always best at, as well as I can. Do I want to play ladies' doubles on a cobbled-together team and then sit down with the other players to eat cake and sandwiches afterward? Sort of. I mean, I definitely did when I started. Only two months ago I drove all the way to Bromley for my first-ever league match with a terrified partner—Netball Hannah— who admitted she was only really interested in the afternoon tea. When I started playing tennis again, only last July, the idea of playing in any kind of league felt impossibly thrilling. Like publishing a book (if you haven't), or becoming a professor. Now what I want to know is which league, and with whom, and will the results affect my rating and my ranking? And I'd much rather it was singles than doubles. And if everyone could please, please just take it a bit more seriously . . .

Today I'm playing with Schoolteacher Hannah (different from Netball Hannah). We are playing Gemma and Linda from Somewhere-Near-Rochester. They are good but have not warmed up and are not used to this surface. We take the first set quite easily. I am nervous, of course, but also Gemma is so oddly beautiful that

I'm having trouble concentrating. She has dark, shiny hair, piercing blue eyes, and a straight nose. Will this sound weird? Here goes anyway: She looks a bit like me. Perhaps fifteen years ago when I was younger, thinner, and prettier. She is wearing a proper tennis outfit—matching top and skirt. Everyone else apart from us is just wearing mismatched tracksuit bottoms and any old top, but she looks as if she has dressed up for this. Her arms are nicer than mine. She has a more beautiful forehand, which she plays early and with plenty of topspin. Oh, and she does that little kick with her right leg as she strikes the ball. She looks quite posh. I am almost falling in love with her—I mean, not *really*, but you know—when we change over before the third set tiebreak. They have just come back from 0–4 down in the second set to take it 6–4. I should stop looking at Gemma. I should hit the ball harder and more aggressively. I should stop thinking and let myself play . . .

This is when Hannah admits, to all of us, to sharing a bottle of wine with her husband last night and I, rather against what I think would be Brad Gilbert's advice, admit to doing the same with my partner. It seems Linda has similarly indulged. But then Gemma pipes up, in a voice that certainly does not match her outfit, "I done *two* bottles of wine with my boyfriend last night."

After this, of course they beat us. It is genius. It is beyond Brad. I am gutted. Then we beat the other pair 6–0, 6–0 and feel a bit better. Then we all sit down to have what's left of the tea and Hannah tells me all about how she had to go to the back of beyond the week before to play with someone named Lucille who was apparently so good that everyone complained. I want to be so good that everyone—in fact, just one person would be fine—complains. But I am not that good. I was a child prodigy, sort of, but I have not played for years and years. I am trying to pick up where I left off on a remote school tennis court back in 1986, when I had hair like Madonna and an accent not unlike Gemma's.

More pictures of the puppy are going around.

It is January 11, 2014. This, I have decided, is going to be my year of tennis. I am going to see how far I can get as a forty-one-year-old woman tennis player, and I'm going to write about it. It's my new project. My new life.

•

Since I've started playing tennis again, I have realized that very few people play singles. It's too hard, too intense. The local leagues only offer doubles matches. People are impressed when I tell them that I play league tennis, but I know the truth—doubles is for fat losers who can't run. The next—and as far as I know only— local singles tournament is the Indoor Tennis Centre Spring Tournament. It's different from the Christmas one. It's rated as a Grade 4 on the LTA website, which means it's county standard. That means that the person most likely to win it will be a county-level player, not me.

You sign up for the tournament on the LTA website. You need a BTM—British Tennis Membership—number to enter proper tournaments like this one. I should have a BTM number, and should have provided it at the few league doubles matches I have already played. I have filled out a form and Margaret has sent it somewhere. Nothing has happened. I have chased it, only to be told that these things are sometimes slow but it will come through eventually. Without the number I can browse tournaments on the LTA website but cannot enter any. I also cannot have a rating or a ranking. At this moment all I want in life is a rating and a ranking. I want numbers that tell me how good a tennis player I am, and then I want to devote my waking life—and maybe even my dreams too—into making those numbers better. I can get a BTM myself, instantly, by paying £25 on the LTA website. But I am not to do this, I am told, because if I just wait I can have the number for free.

And then one night I do it. Of course I do. It's probably the best £25 I have ever spent. It means I can turn my life into a sort of video game. *And fuck*, I suddenly think, *all those stupid years I spent playing video games because they were cheap and easy when I could have been doing this.* I was younger and my muscles were looser and my reactions were faster but of course I had no money for shoes or lessons, and instead I had all those deadlines and panic attacks and cigarettes. Breathe. Yes, OK, though, the thing I did like about video games is also the thing I like about this. I am going to get a rating and then I am going to play other people with ratings and I am going to win or lose and my rating is going to go up or down and between matches I will power up and learn special skills and work on my sword and . . .

And I can enter the Spring Tournament. I will have my own "competition calendar." I can't remember the last time I was this excited about anything. Speaking in front of five hundred people at the Sydney Writers' Festival last year, I just wished it would be over so I could go and eat oysters and drink wine, but things are different this year. This year I am going to be fierce and thin and a champion. But when I go on to the LTA website to enter the Spring Tournament, it tells me that I can't enter online and have to do it at the tennis center. So I have to sheepishly admit to Margaret that I paid £25 to join the LTA—which I don't mind, I stress, I *don't mind at all*—but that it won't let me enter the tournament. While she waits for the website to load so she can check what's gone wrong, because you should be able to enter online, should be able to put the tournament in your "shopping basket" as if it were just another strategy book or sports bra from Amazon, I ask if it's going to be another round robin like the Christmas Tournament. It can't be, Margaret explains, because she is expecting around eighty people to enter. I guess that's men and kids as well as women. But even so . . .

"It'll be knockout, probably," she says.

"So there'll be like a draw, and seeds, and—"

"And a consolation draw," she says. "So everyone who comes can play at least two games. I mean, otherwise it's unfair on someone who draws the top seed in the first round."

But what if that was me? How badly would the top seed in a Level 4 tournament beat me? Would it be bagels? Or would I— *could* I—beat her? What if one day I *was* her? Or am I supposed to just accept that now, at forty-one, I am never going to be a top seed, nor beat one? At this stage I have literally no concept of what a good player actually is. My life experience of sport so far has been scattered and inconsistent and largely free of any experience leading to hard knocks leading to actual knowledge. All I have are vague memories of my mother telling me I was good enough for Wimbledon. Being proud of those few points I took off Couze. The Middlesex thing. Oh, God, the Middlesex thing. And still, in this already aging millennium, *still* this feeling of if you want something badly enough and if you train for it and pray for it and, yes, pay for it, then it can be yours—anything, *anything* you want so long as you want it badly enough—and as yet I have absolutely no idea, no fucking idea that every single tennis parent and middle-aged wannabe in the whole country feels exactly the same way.

•

I was fourteen when I gave up tennis. It was 1986.

I'd gone to boarding school, which was where it happened. How to tell this story, which in itself is sort of like my whole life story? It was my dad who sent me to boarding school, but only after my other dad had gone to America to marry an heiress and begin the heroin habit that would slowly kill him. I'd only known who my "real" father was for a couple of years. Mum had had an affair, romantic and beautiful and tragic, with this tousle-haired, Gauloise-smoking, blue-eyed, Serge Gainsbourg look-alike back in the early 1970s. I was the result, in 1972. He was called Gordian, like the knot. He had a complicated, rich, Jewish mother, who'd escaped Hitler by riding a bicycle from Luxembourg to France. He had a beautiful, cool, tap-dancing sister. Mum's then husband Steve agreed to bring me up as his own, but Gordian came to visit every week, when he wasn't in the midst of a cocaine overdose or Valium meltdown or anxiety attack. Ten years or so later Mum had another affair, this time with her university lecturer, Couze, and one day we went to live with him and everything changed. It wasn't long after that when I played tennis for the first time.

But for now, let's skip to the last time.

I was good. Good enough that I'd been asked to play for Middlesex, or maybe train with them, or maybe just try out for them, back in 1984, during my first tennis holiday at the David Lloyd Centre in Hounslow. I couldn't do it, of course, because we lived miles away, but still. In 1986 I was just back from another solo holiday, this time all the way to Mexico to stay with my new grandmother, Ruth, who wore caftans, made tuna mousse in smoked-glass bowls, and was obsessed with a flamboyant gay man named Patricio.

Say what you like about the posh European half of my gene pool, but they know how to do things properly. When the trip was being planned, I was asked what activities I did. Horse-riding (which Gordian had rediscovered in the '80s rather as I have resumed tennis now) and, of course, tennis. So I had to take a riding hat and a racquet. There was to be some horse-riding with local children and—joy—tennis coaching several afternoons a week. The coaching was amazing. Hot, dripping hot, with fresh orange juice afterward, and sometimes spicy Mexican food. And I was good, hitting hard back and forth with the coach for a whole sun-drenched hour. Crosscourt forehands. Crosscourt backhands. Forehands down the line. Backhands down the line. Serving. Volleying. Points. I remember the coach commenting on my ability, perhaps asking me what club or team I played for back at home. Was I a player *nationale*, or *regionale*? But at home there was no national, regional, or even local club or team, never had been.

Why? I still don't know.

Back at home the miners had finished striking, but Nelson Mandela was yet to be released. In 1987 a lot of our family energy would go into trying to get Neil Kinnock elected prime minister. We were always doing things to try to undermine Thatcher, like watching *Spitting Image* and going on demonstrations against whatever she was doing, whether it was closing pits, canceling free milk for schoolchildren, or inventing the new poll tax. Home was about trying to fit in at my local school, where girls my age were into horses and boys and no one played tennis. No one played any sport, not really, apart from football perhaps, but this was before the Premier League, when it was still muddy and real and sort of for thickos. Otherwise, sport was clean and healthy and airy but clearly for simple people who *did not care* that the world was gray and hard and full of poverty and racism and fascism and about to be nuked anyway.

And there was nowhere to play tennis most of the time. The

grass courts near our house in Chelmsford had weeds growing on them year-round. The concrete courts were better, but some council official took the nets away in October and didn't put them up again until April. I dreaded Wimbledon; at that time all it meant to me was that the tennis courts—my tennis courts—would be full for two weeks while people tried out their McEnroe moves or in some way tried to emulate whoever they'd just been watching on their tiny, possibly still black-and-white TVs. And playing tennis was expensive, perhaps £1.50 an hour. Although Couze and I always tried to dodge the inspector, we had to pay up if he did come round. It was also a treat, of course, and treats needed to be rationed, and I had homework to do and my brother to look after and given that the world was surely going to end when the US bombed the USSR . . . The only indoor tennis center I knew was in Hounslow, a good couple of hours away on the other side of London. The only coaches I knew were there too. Too far. Too hard. Too posh. Too exclusive. Not for the likes of us.

Tennis was my first love. Every other sport I ever played was with my eyes closed and the duvet stuffed in my mouth so I didn't shout out its name, the name of my real passion, my soulmate.

Tennis.

Which I let go so easily. Which I just *dropped*. Why?

Here is what I remember. The Troellers—Grandmother Ruth and Gordian—decided to send me to boarding school. Or maybe my mother decided I should go to a private school and got them to pay for it. But that's unlikely, since we were such devoted lefties who were, of course, quite against private education. So let's say the Troellers decided. It was just after I came back from Mexico, after all. Ruth had found me common, as well as uncouth and unsophisticated and weird, with my Walkman, my Madonna hair, my turquoise espadrilles. She would talk seriously about my coming out, not as a lesbian but as a debutante, and she assumed my family owned a fax machine and that I would apply to study philosophy, politics, and economics at Oxford or law at Cambridge. She was so elitist and stuck-up and posh! In a world where all good people were striving for equality and justice, she threw cocktail parties and insisted on reading *Class* by Jilly Cooper, not just to herself but out loud to me. I mean, it was funny, of course, but totally wrong. Gordian thought my school friends were common. They were! So was I, a bit. Or I wanted to be. At that time, I actually did want to be named Sharon or Tracey and live on a council estate and eat chips every night and drink Nesquik.

So they sent me to boarding school.

And that was where it happened. Again, my memory is hazy. I remember a hard outdoor tennis court and possibly some weak autumn sunshine. Was it the first time I'd played on these courts? Possibly. Why were we playing tennis in autumn? Who knows? Maybe it didn't happen until the spring term, or even the summer term. I was having trouble fitting into my new school, full of mini Grandmother Ruths who assumed everyone voted Conservative and who talked of "plebs" and—worse—village boys, also known as VBs. The big thing at my boarding school was lacrosse, known as "lax." The most popular girl in the form, Kate, and her sidekick Danielle, regularly played in the school's second XI. Given that they both smoked, and were only in the fourth form, this was a big achievement. Kate was sometimes bumped up to the First Team. It was unspeakably glamorous.

Again, no one played tennis. Was that the problem? Or was it rather that *everyone* played tennis? Half of them probably had courts in their gardens at home and found the whole thing a big yawn, maybe something to do lazily with a brother or cousin on a summer's afternoon. But here's the dreadful thing: They were good at it. Good enough for me not to seem like a child prodigy, not to shine, not to dazzle. Especially since, on that afternoon, my first time playing tennis at this school, I was playing so badly.

What was the teacher doing? Perhaps something I found patronizing. Perhaps something I just thought was wrong. Perhaps we were doing lame, babyish forehand drills. Perhaps she had told me to grip my racquet differently, assuming I was a mere mortal, a simple child who hadn't played much before. I hate being told what to do and always think I know best. This was true even when I was a fourteen-year-old outsider at a new school. Still, I now don't remember exactly what was wrong with the lesson. What I do remember is that I choked. I froze. I got the Elbow. Just like Eugenie Bouchard in the first set of the Australian Open semifinal in 2014. Of course in that case the commentators knew what it was. She needed to settle down, breathe, relax into the match, they said. And by the time I watched that match I knew all about choking too, or thought I did, and had half a dozen books that addressed the subject and offered remedies for it. Not that any of them ever really worked.

But back in 1986 I didn't know what was happening to me. I had no idea that this was a phenomenon, a thing that happens when you are nervous, when you desperately want to play well or win or show someone how good you are. I played one of the other girls, I can't remember who, but I'm pretty sure she was not any kind of tennis prodigy. And she beat me. I didn't even have to give her any points. I'm fairly sure that's what happened, although I have no real memory of it, just the feeling of choking and being beaten and not being at all special.

And I gave up tennis. Whatever actually happened, I remember being there on those courts and feeling that I'd been wrong all along. Out there in the world of plebs? Yes, perhaps there I was good at tennis, but here everything was different. In this new world, this new life, for which I had even renamed myself Victoria—my middle name—because I was sick of having to explain Scarlett, I was not good at tennis. I was just average. My dream, such as it was, was over. When it came to choosing extracurricular activities I picked ballet and horse-riding. And for the rest of the time I threw myself into learning lacrosse, and how to smoke, and how to be good at dieting.

•

2014. It's a murky January day and I'm having lunch on the seafront with David Flusfeder. The day before, my picture appeared in the local newspaper. In the picture I'm holding both my tennis trophies from the Christmas Tournament—the one they let me take home and the one that stays in the tennis center—and I look really, genuinely happy. I tell him that I have only won one trophy in my life before, a blocky, Lucite Elle Style Award for my novel *Going Out*. I remember feeling how random that all was and how winning was all down to the whims of the judges. I couldn't bring myself to go to the ceremony because I didn't have anything to wear and I vaguely disapproved of anything A-listy, so I made my long-suffering agent Simon go instead. I was longlisted for the Orange Prize for Fiction in 2008 but couldn't do anything to get myself onto the shortlist. With tennis you train and then turn up with your racquets and your bag full of stuff and you win or lose points that everyone agrees on, that exist in the world and not just in someone's head. I have recently realized that I am prouder of my small, cheap tennis trophy than almost anything else in my life.

"So I'm really going to go for it this year," I tell David. "I'm going to totally throw myself into tennis and see how far I can get. I mean, I'm going to enter actual singles tournaments and have massages and stay in hotels and everything."

I wonder if he's going to laugh at me but instead he makes interested, even encouraging noises. I tell him I might even write a book about it, because that'll give me an excuse to really do it properly—and, in the tradition of all such projects, take semi-stupid risks and embarrass myself in the name of research and "just write down what happens." I explain that if I lose everything and look stupid then that'll make quite a funny book, and if I win everything and feel amazing the book won't be so good but who cares—I'd rather have another trophy than another book anyway. I didn't realize then that there was a third, awful, option. I had no idea.

"You're having coaching?"

"Yeah. Of course."

"Have more. Do everything you can to win."

"Sadly, I think 'more' is sort of frowned on."

"Why? By whom?"

"The other people who go to the tennis center. People believe that you shouldn't buy success. They're always saying to me things like, 'Wow, you're really coming on. Dan must be an amazing coach.' It's like he's the one who's done it, not me, and anyone rich and stupid enough to fork out £25 a week on coaching would become as good as me."

"That's ridiculous."

"I know. I mean it is, but also I think it's because I'm basically a middle-aged woman, and what kind of middle-aged woman invests time and money in sport for herself and not for her son or daughter or whatever? I mean, what kind of woman seriously takes up a sport again at forty-one and then expects to actually go somewhere with it? I do worry that people are basically laughing at me."

"Forget what these people think. Stop worrying about people judging you. You've got to go all-out to win and just don't think about it. Get more coaching. Get as much coaching as you can possibly afford."

•

Princess Helena College, 1987. We are not allowed to watch TV during the week, and can only watch a limited amount during the weekend where we have to sit around together—the whole fifth form, except for Claire Bolton, who will be practicing playing Chopin somewhere else—and watch something approved by the teachers. Mostly it is videos, and my fifth form is a blur of *Footloose* and *Flashdance* and other PG-13 films about finding yourself through dance and convincing the establishment that being young and taking risks is better than being old and boring and conservative.

My very favorite of all the films we watch is *Dirty Dancing*. Jennifer Grey's character, known as Baby but actually named Frances, is going with her parents and sister to a holiday camp where rich chicks pay for dance lessons with hot young dudes. Desperate to be authentic and accepted, one night Baby makes her way to the staff quarters and sees them doing their real dancing—dirty dancing—not nice dancing, the inauthentic crap they have to do with the wrinkled, loaded, old women who have to pay to be looked at, touched, taken seriously. Jennifer Grey is thin, so thin. She is beautiful and misunderstood and intelligent. The hottest guy in the whole thing, dance instructor Johnny Castle, played by Patrick Swayze, is a working-class hero with a sassy, seen-it-all dance partner, Penny. They do the major shows together for the lamest tourists with the biggest bucks, but then it turns out that Penny is pregnant, and idealistic Baby wants to help—even though in the real world sometimes you can't help—and gets her doctor father to save Penny after a botched abortion almost kills her. Now Patrick Swayze has no dance partner for a big show and no one can fill in for Penny because they all *work*, remember, unlike the lazy, rich holidaymakers. (It wasn't Johnny who got Penny pregnant, by the way. We learn to be very suspicious about the easy assumptions the idiotic rich make about the noble poor.)

But the thing is, Baby does it.

She learns to dance, from scratch, so she can fill in for Penny.

I have only recently realized that I probably ended up basing my life on this film. I've always loved stories of hard work and miracles and anything being possible if you only try. As a kid, one of my favorite books was *Tony's Hard Work Day*, which tells of a four-year-old boy who is not allowed to help repair his family's new house because he is too small. What does Tony do? He goes off on his own and builds a whole new house! In a day! It's such a good house that his family immediately abandons their old house and moves straight in.

But *Dirty Dancing* wasn't just about Baby overcoming the odds to become a professional-standard dancer in just a few days. It was about her being *chosen* to do it, singled out, made special. OK, we are supposed to believe that she has no ability and that all she really has in her favor is time, because she is on holiday. At fifteen I just took it for granted that she was hot and young and thin. I was too, and so were my friends. All we needed was to find ourselves in a situation like that.

One scene shows Baby discovering that Johnny Castle doesn't

just teach dancing to the withered, alcoholic, over-made-up old crones at the holiday camp. He does *extras* too. Baby freaks out, of course, only to be told to grow up, because this is the real world. When I first watched this scene, surrounded by my rich, beautiful schoolfriends, all I saw was Baby, her lack of worldliness, her desire to be grown up. I saw myself in her. I'd never had a job, had only just started experimenting with black eyeliner, was still (just) a virgin. I simply did not notice the older women in the film, let alone imagine I could ever become them. Perhaps you're not supposed to. As well as the crone who has to pay to be fucked, there's the wife who doesn't really understand the husband, and of course the many other recipients of Johnny Castle's dance lessons, and they are all old and disgusting and they play it safe and don't take risks and would never, ever be asked to fill in as anyone's dance partner.

•

It's a rainy Thursday in October 2013, and I turn up for my coaching session in even more strapping than usual. My knees are both so sore that I have ordered a new knee brace so I can wear two at once. I can hardly walk down the stairs. What the fuck am I doing playing tennis? But I've had three ibuprofen. I'm sure when they kick in I'll be fine. Dan is at the reception desk when I arrive, joking around with the staff. Everyone is giggling, happy. Dan has this effect on people.

"What are you doing tonight?" he asks me.

"Why? I mean, nothing, but why?"

"Good. You're playing tennis with me. I need a doubles partner."

"OK." *Breathe. Don't die. Breathe.* "My knees are a bit crap at the moment."

"That's OK. I'll do all the running for you. 7:00 p.m.?"

I am so happy I could vomit. Immediately a voice in my head points out that this is quite short notice and he has probably asked literally everyone else in the entire world, but it's only 2:00 p.m. The match isn't until 7:00 p.m. There are five hours' worth of people he has not yet asked. This is one of the best, most exciting things that has ever happened to me. Dan thinks I'm good enough to play in a league doubles match with him. Oh, God. Oh, God.

The coaching session that follows is the best I've ever had. I'm hitting the ball hard and deep but keeping it in. A couple of my crosscourt shots are so good that Dan makes a kind of whistling noise. He hardly ever praises me. I feel amazing. He has me on the forehand side hitting crosscourt into the tramlines, because I'll be playing forehand tonight. I am in training for something! It is real. I keep playing better than I ever have before. After the session is over, I rush home and tell Rod what has happened. I have a bath. Stretch. Eat scrambled eggs. I am so nervous I feel a bit sick. Apart from Bromley, I have never played a league match before.

We hit up with other members of our team. I feel like I am fifteen years old and trying to buy something cool from the Our Price record store in Chelmsford. Walking feels strange. Speaking feels strange. The others seem so relaxed, but I keep netting the ball or hitting it to the wrong side of the court. I'm sure it will stop when we begin playing, but it doesn't. It gets worse. I am a disaster. An embarrassment. Why did I think I could do this? I fluff most of my shots, but Dan rescues the whole thing and we somehow win our first match, 6–3, 6–3.

"It should have been love and love," he tells me in the break.

I take a deep breath. "Look, I'm really sorry I'm so nervous and . . ."

"You'll be all right," he says, not quite making eye contact.

The next pair are much better. The man intercepts at the net. It's hard to get anything past him. Still, since we've won the first match, I've relaxed quite a lot. I even manage to hit a nice shot down the tramlines behind the man when he moves the other way to poach a ball he thinks is coming crosscourt.

"Shot!" says Dan. We fist-bump. This is fun, suddenly.

The ball comes to me on the forehand side. I hit a good lob over the volleyer. The server, the woman, has to run to her backhand side and try to get it back, but her shot is weak and it's a very, very easy overhead for Dan to just . . .

Put straight in the net.

WTF? To me Dan is the Best Tennis Player Ever, but in this match he makes more and more errors. My confidence is going up and so, apparently, is his, but every serve he goes for is intended to be an ace. In one game he double-faults three times. He tries to poach at the net and misses. I can tell he's tired. I guess he's been coaching all day. He's playing on the ad side, the left, because in doubles the strongest player always goes on the ad side. During one long deuce, though, I notice we are getting to advantage on my point and then back to deuce on his. Am I playing *better* than Dan? If so it's only for a few minutes, but . . . I'm not exactly keeping track of the score but I know I'm suddenly enjoying this. Dan and I have never played together before and we won our first match and we're doing OK against good opponents in this one. We fight for the first set but lose 6–4. That's OK, right? We lose the next one 6–2.

Dan lies on the ground afterward, not meeting my eye.

OK. So.

He keeps lying there. I put my stuff away. He goes to the office.

When I get home I feel low, childish, sour. I tell Rod all about the matches and how well I played toward the end, but when I try to tell him how upset I am because Dan didn't say anything to me afterward, he doesn't get it. Maybe Dan was tired? Undoubtedly. He could have said thanks, though. He could have said I did well in my very first mixed doubles match ever. He's my coach, right? I feel miserable all weekend. On Monday evening I go along to the club night that Dan runs.

"You know," I say to him, "that was the first time I have ever played mixed doubles in my life. I mean in an actual match. And—"

He's bounding along with a basket of balls.

"Well, you're playing again on Thursday," he says.

•

I recently left my literary agent. He was a nice person, a good friend. We used to go to polite places and I would drink wine while he had sparkling mineral water and talked about training for marathons. My new agent goes around in an anorak clutching grubby, suspicious-looking bags of books and vaguely menacing all the people who bother him on the Tube. He meets his authors in a variety of terrible dives ranging from YO! Sushi to sticky Soho pubs. He is always late. I once invited him for afternoon tea. "Tea? I do not drink *tea*," was the response. He is one of the best readers I have ever encountered and represents all the most exciting authors in the UK, even though some of them remain so poor that they plead with him to get them in prison.

I'm not sure whether moving to him was the right choice, but it's too late now. I did it on a whim. My long-term agent had taken too long to reply to an email and so I did one of those things I now often do when I'm angry: something random and unkind and completely undoable. I DMed David Miller on Twitter and suggested a coffee.

We met at Paddington station and I felt like I was embarking on an affair and I didn't care.

It's January 2014. I have recently delivered my new novel and so we are meeting for dinner. Because I live in Kent and David is based in London, he has suggested meeting at a halfway point, in Ashford, where another of his authors set one of her novels. "No," I'd said. "They have no wine in Ashford. And no food." I'm still quite into wine and food. I suggest meeting in Blacks, my private members club in Soho. My current favorite wine at Blacks is called Cunto and costs £42 a bottle.

"Where does your train come in? St. Pancras?"

He knows a pub near St. Pancras, although "near" turns out to be over the other side of Kings Cross toward the *Guardian* building. It's cold and raining, and this is too short a distance to get a cab or a Tube. The pub is busy but at least the wine is OK. David is forty minutes late, which means I have one glass of wine and then another and another. We walk in the rain to a restaurant on the Euston Road where the most expensive bottle of wine is £12.99 and everything comes with fries. I'm tired from work and tennis and a bit drunk. We should have gone to Ashford, but it's too late. David wants to talk about the novel I've just delivered. He says he thinks it is all about love, which is true: it is. But I can't get properly in the mood. In fact, I suddenly want to tell him about something different. I take out my iPad and bring up the piece about the Christmas Tournament from the *East Kent Mercury*. There's a picture of me holding my trophy next to pictures of Amie Tonkiss and her father with their doubles trophy. I'm smiling broadly. My hair is scraped back. I'm wearing my best Stella McCartney white warm-up jacket, and I'm pleased that I remembered to put lipstick on for the photo.

David scans the piece. There is no expression on his face. Then he laughs.

"Hilarious that there's another Scarlett Thomas in East Kent," he says.

"That's me," I say.

"What?"

"That's me."

"That's not you. You've got cheekbones."

I roll my eyes. "I was playing sport. With my hair up."

He takes my iPad again. Scrutinizes the story more closely.

"Look," I say, waving my fingers. "Same color nail polish."

He frowns. "But your face is so fat in this picture."

I roll my eyes again. "OK. Look, I won this trophy last month. I'm forty-one. I think I could have been a great tennis player but I had nowhere to play seriously when I was a kid. Basically, I'm going to write a tennis book. I'm going to spend 2014 playing tennis and I'm going to see how far I can get. In a year. As a forty-one-year-old. And I'm going to find out whether I would rather have been a tennis player than a novelist—"

He nods. Sighs. "All right," he says. "OK. How far could you go?"

"Sorry? What, do you mean like in tournaments?"

"Could you, in theory, get to Wimbledon?"

"In a year, no. At my age, no. In theory, though, yes. Sort of."

"You *could* get to Wimbledon?"

"Anyone could get to Wimbledon. It's one of the good things about the LTA system. If I went out now and just won all my matches, eventually my rating would get higher and then I'd get into better tournaments and eventually, yes, there's no reason—well, apart from all the obvious ones—why anyone couldn't get to Wimbledon."

Like Baby with her dancing, and four-year-old Tony with his house.

"Anyway, I'm going to get massages and stay in places like the Leicester Hilton and, I don't know, try to see a part of the world that most people don't get to see. Are there other fortysomething women out there trying to do sport at a high level? Who are they? What are they like? And what about me? Can I do it? What will it feel like to win?"

David frowns. "Travelodge," he says.

"What? No way, I'm—"

"It'll be a far better story if you stay in a Travelodge."

•

Did I really never play tennis in all those years, between giving it up at fourteen and taking it up again at forty-one? Of course I played. There was always a racquet in the back of a cupboard, and always a new boyfriend to beat. I could beat people, even in those wilderness years, because I am fast and good with a ball, and something of those coaching sessions in Mexico stayed with me forever. But it was nowhere near enough. There was the day when a good friend whose major flaw was misogyny (which didn't apply to me, of course, just all other women) told me of a fight he'd had with his soon-to-be ex-wife, where he'd said that any man could beat any woman at tennis, and she'd said all right then, let's play, and he'd gone out and thrashed her. He said she'd deserved it. *Come on then*, I'd said, *I'll beat you now*. And I did. With horrible shots and underspin—underspin!—but really just by being able to play the ball in places where he wasn't. The ball would come and I would visualize what I wanted to do with it, and then it would go out or in the net. But I still got more points than he did.

In 2007 I had a bestseller for the first time and so I took my mum on holiday to Gozo. After a few days I got bored lying around in the sun (and felt fat, always worried about feeling fat) and I so desperately wanted to run, I wanted to hit something, I wanted that thrill of competing, even if not in a real competition. So I booked a coach and got a really shit racquet from behind the hotel desk. I wore a beach wrap and espadrilles. I looked utterly ridiculous. I didn't care. *You could be quite good*, the coach said in broken English. *Let me show you how to* . . . But I didn't want to be shown how to. In these precious sixty minutes, dwindling all the time to fifty-nine, fifty-eight, fifty-seven, just like life, ticking down, receding, all I wanted to do was play tennis. I just wanted to hit the ball. I didn't care how.

When I got back from Gozo I joined the Canterbury Tennis Club. I could afford it, and the £25 Slazenger racquet that I later used for my first session with Dan. After my first mix-in session, the best player there wanted to chat with me. I'd played a couple of—I'll say so myself—pretty awesome shots as part of my rusty, slightly humiliating performance, and assumed that he wanted to talk to me about that. But no, he just wanted to show me his photographs, which became more explicit once all the other players left. When I realized I was on my own at the wrong end of a sports club in the rangy Kent countryside, with this guy showing me pictures of a woman who was by then not only topless but bottomless too, I left and never went back. I wasn't so upset about the photographs—it wasn't the first time this kind of thing had happened to me—but more that my shots were so crap. I would never, ever get back whatever it was I'd had as a kid, that I maybe never even had anyway. It was really over this time.

•

January 2014. It's less than two weeks until my Leicester tournament. My train tickets have arrived. I have booked a room in the Leicester Hilton, which has a gym, swimming pool, and sauna. I've been stalking my opponents on the LTA website, finding out what year they were born and what other tournaments they've played. This is not helping at all. Someone I could play against has a national ranking of thirteenth in her age group. What will it be like actually playing one of these people? I start planning my coaching and hitting sessions for the week beforehand. I am organized, focused. I send an email to the tournament organizer asking if he can put me in touch with any local coaches so I can have a hit on the surface for an hour before the tournament begins. He sends me the number of someone named Dave. Before I leave, I particularly want the ball machine for a couple of hours on Sunday, but the courts in the Indoor Tennis Centre are all booked up for tournaments and matches.

"But since you're free on Sunday," begins Margaret.

This time I have to bring cold meats.

We are playing Bearsted IV. They turn up grumpy from the journey and wet from the storm outside. They are wearing fleeces that say things like MAIDSTONE HARRIERS or simply BEARSTED LTC. The whole thing is supposed to begin at 2:30 but there is a kids' mini-tournament that's running over and, on Courts 3 and 4, the *slap, slap, thwack* of two regional boys' under-16 semifinals. I've already been down that end of the tennis center by accident and I watched the boys for a few minutes before the umpire glared at me and made it clear I should leave. These boys play the kind of tennis I want to play. They serve hard, wallop the ball around the court, and fling their tennis racquets at the wall when they make a mistake. They are focused. They are grunting. One of them does it loud, like Nadal. He is beautiful.

I have my period. And a hangover.

Bearsted IV are being passive-aggressive about the time delay. They let us know that even though they are not enforcing a penalty (which I think might be a set in their favor), they could. Despite the period and the hangover, I have been to the gym and warmed up as usual. Five minutes on the bike followed by twenty minutes of stretches and running on the spot and pretending to be Victoria Azarenka. But now, in the vast unheated space of the Indoor Tennis Centre, I am freezing again. Margaret is trying to free up another court. When we do eventually get Court 3, we are delayed further because the nets are set up for singles rather than doubles. Once we take down the singles sticks, the net sags to a ridiculously low height. Hannah and I start trying to find both the winding thing for making the net go up and down and the measuring stick to make the net the right height.

Bearsted IV's first pair are tutting and sighing. I have period pains. I am now on six ibuprofen a day pretty much every day, because if it's not period pains it's my knees or my lower back. We get the net the right height. I arrange the chairs and get out my small pink Lucozade and my large Evian and consider pointing them at the court like Nadal does, but don't. We begin hitting up. I tell myself to touch my back with my racquet as I finish each forehand. To leave space between me and the ball. I pose like the Statue of Liberty after each backhand. They have won the toss and decided to serve. Their serve is by far the weakest aspect of their game, but a lot of people choose to serve first just because it is what big men with big serves do. It is what Pete Sampras would have done. We take the first game easily.

I am serving next. Last time I played Dan I really worked on my serve, trying to outthink him, trying to make something happen. In the heat of contest, I developed a lovely new serve out wide to the backhand on the ad court, but I can't serve that here because Hannah's head is in the way. In doubles there is always someone or some part of someone in the way. It is one of the things I most hate about it. I have never really bothered to work on that doubles serve where you go out really wide to get the angles. I usually just aim for the T and try to baffle the opposition with a choice of two serves: spin or no spin. Anyway, today my serve has deserted me. In one game we get stuck on deuce for about thirty-five minutes. Hannah has to get back to Sandwich for a dinner party at 6:00 p.m. We begin to worry. But then my serve comes back and we win the first set easily, 6–2.

I am volleying well, feeling confident and happy at the net. I even play a couple of really good overheads. I am fast and aggressive, but my ground stroke game feels wrong. I just keep plonking it back to the baseline player and trying to avoid the one at the net. And they have clearly decided to step it up in this set. They match us game for game until we break them and I serve for the match on 5–4. I find I am horribly nervous through the two match points that we lose, one to a double fault. I keep thinking *This is match point*, and it doesn't help. We lose my service game, which means we've gone from match point to having to win another two games to take the set 5–7. But this doesn't happen. Instead, we end up on a tiebreak at 6–6.

Kent Slazenger Inter Club Leagues matches are decided on the best of three sets, but the third set is always a championship tiebreak, which is first to ten points. This means that if we lose one tiebreak, we will have to play another immediately. And after we lost two match points! If Bearsted IV's first pair win one tiebreak, the momentum will go with them and we will lose the next one as well. This dreadful thought stays with me until we are 0–5 down and I decide to do something about it. I'm not sure exactly what changes. I hate losing; I think that is the main thing. Suddenly I am much more aggressive. I am following everything I play into the net and swatting away the returns. Hannah is playing well too. We are particularly good with her keeping it steady at the back and me slamming them away at the front. We make it to 5–5 and all the momentum is back with us. They win one more point but we take the tiebreak 8–6 and the set 7–6 and the match 2–0.

Our other pair have beaten their other pair easily and have been sitting around in the cold for about an hour, watching us play. Bearsted's other pair are also cold. And bored. And hungry. One of them is a woman of about my age. The other looks like a picture-book granny. She has a gray perm and a velour tracksuit the color of an inflamed hemorrhoid. I am toweling down after finishing our first match and preparing to move my stuff to Court 2. It is customary, and polite, to let the away team stay on their courts.

"Have you got a biscuit or something, love?" asks the older woman.

"Sorry?" I say.

"It's just that it's ever so late, and we've been waiting ever such a long time."

"Um."

"I think I might be feeling a bit dizzy. It's just so late, and—"

"I've got a Dairy Milk you can have if you like," I offer. I always have spare Cadbury Dairy Milks. I'm not sure that giving one to the opposition would be something Brad Gilbert would approve of, but

I feel sorry for this poor old woman who is clearly unable to walk to the other side of the room and get a chocolate bar from the machine. Or, in the long wait she has just had, to discover the café upstairs.

"Oh no, dear. Not if it's out of your own personal supply. What's that under there?" She points under Hannah's chair to a Sainsbury's carrier bag filled with cake.

"Cake," I say. "For afternoon tea. But I haven't got a knife to cut it with. Are you sure you don't just want a Dairy Milk?"

"You shouldn't have to give us something of your own."

"But we buy the cake anyway. And, in fact, the whole afternoon tea. So it's pretty much all 'our own.'"

"I only want a biscuit."

"OK, well, I'm sorry, but we just don't have any biscuits."

"I had a banana at lunch time, but now I just feel a bit dizzy, and ..."

For goodness' sake. If you want biscuits that much, surely you bring your own? I wouldn't dream of going anywhere to play tennis without at least 1.5 liters of water and several Dairy Milks just in case. You never know what you're going to find when you go somewhere to play tennis. Although look at me, who has only ever made it to one away game ever. But if even I know this, you'd think that this old bird, who has clearly been around the block a few times, would remember to stick some cookies in her bloody handbag.

Hannah and I don't exactly say it, but we know we are about to double-bagel these two. It's now 5:00 p.m. We agree that we'll have this match finished within an hour. Improbably, though, Bearsted IV's second pair win the first game. Neither moves her feet much; the older lady not at all. The younger woman plays every forehand with the kind of underspin I last saw in Central Park, Chelmsford, Essex, in the 1980s. The older woman plonks everything. Whatever you hit to her she plonks back with an accuracy that quickly becomes unnerving. These two also love lobbing. And volleying. Anything that involves standing still they do really well. I don't mean that in an entirely disparaging way; after all, it's working. A couple of times Hannah waits for the underspin forehand to bounce so she can get a really good swing at it, only to find she is swinging the wrong way and the sneaky little thing has crept under her racquet. In West Indian cricket I believe a similar ball is called a rat.

On the first game changeover, I go to update the score. Every court has its own small scoreboard on a stick with numbers you flip over. The first time I played with Dan I was impressed by how properly he did everything, including keeping the score updated. When it doesn't seem appropriate to pretend I am Azarenka, Serena, Sharapova, Federer, or Nadal, I sometimes pretend I am Dan. Apart from anything else, updating the scoreboard helps passing spectators know what's going on. But it's useful for everyone to know the score. And it shows you care. It is just another one of a thousand small things you can do to transcend the mundane, like performing hamstring stretches properly and drinking water on changeovers. But it's also something that other players sometimes resent, because it involves Taking Everything Too Seriously. As I start flipping the numbers over, the older woman comes and literally breathes down my neck. I can smell cookies. Someone must have found some biscuits.

She's got quite a low voice. "You the little scorer then?"

"I'm not sure I'd put it quite like that," I say.

We lose another game. Then another one.

On the next changeover she comes up to me again. "Doing your little scoreboard, are you?"

"I think you've already pointed that out."

When Novak Djokovic played Fabio Fognini in the 2014 Australian Open a few days before this, one of the commentators observed that there is no intimidating tactic that you are not allowed to use against your opponent in tennis. I begin to think that even Fognini could take lessons from this old dear. All he really did was throw his racquet into Novak's court and make a joke about Monte Carlo.

I give up on the scoreboard. I sit with a towel over my head instead.

On the next changeover it's 2–5. Hannah and I keep shaking our heads and saying what a change of pace this is after the last match, and how we need to get used to the deadly underspin, and how when we do it will be fine, but we need a plan before that. On the last changeover I suggested we hit deeper, but it didn't make any difference. Now I suggest we poach more at the net. I don't know if the old woman heard us, but the first time I try it the ball whistles past me down the tramlines.

"Saw what you were trying to do there, dear," she says, chuckling. I almost think I hear her add "with your little tactics." This is awful. This is a tennis nightmare. This is the kind of dream you are grateful to wake up from. Over on Court 4 the under-16 boys are still thwacking away with beauty, grace, style, and power. I think that if one of them were to glance over here now he'd just see a load of old women playing shit tennis. There would be nothing to distinguish me (or Hannah, although I sense this kind of observation would not bother her as it does me) from the others. Should this matter? Probably not. But I know I am a better player than the people who are beating me. I am up on my toes. I am sweating. I have matching sweatbands! Not just that. I am fitter. Stronger. All my strokes are better. So what the fuck is going on?

We lose the set.

In the break Hannah suggests that as we are going to lose this match anyway, we should probably use it to practice our volleys or some other part of our games. *Lose the match.* I gulp. She's right. If we keep playing like this we are actually going to lose the match. And then I realize that if I lose this match, if I lose to a moonballing grandmother who has not even removed her tracksuit top, I will have to give up tennis forever. I have a coach. A personal trainer. Fifteen books on tennis strategy. Why am I not beating these people? It's not as if I am not talented. I mean, I am talented, right? I certainly was when I was a kid. I'm never going to be as good at doubles as I am at singles, but even so. I breathe. Glance over to Court 4. One of the under-16s is flinging his racquet at the wall. He has passion. I should fling my racquet at the wall too, but I don't.

They win another game.

Fuck this. OK. All right. What is the universe trying to tell me here?

And as soon as I ask, I know. *Swing through my shots. Finish with the racquet touching my back. Grunt.* I made a list just last night of the things I would always try to do in competitive situations and not just in practices. I have done none of these things today. When the old biddy plonks the ball to me, I plonk it back. When she moonballs it to one corner, I moonball it back to another corner. Why am I letting her dictate the play? I go to the gym two or three times a week and I lift weights and I get muscles that I then do not use. I have coaching where I learn to hit shots that I also do not use. Why? Why do I freeze so much in matches that I can't hit the ball properly on my ground strokes? It's not even nerves anymore. It's a weird combination of embarrassment, habit, and politeness. After all, if some nice old lady has just hit you a tennis ball, you automatically hit it back. Don't you?

But she isn't that nice, and I've had enough of this. This time when she serves, I attack it. I take my racquet back and swing properly at the ball, pulling the racquet up and over the ball to create as much topspin as I can. I finish with the racquet over my head. I grunt. All these things are slightly staged. I realize I am forcing myself to grunt rather than it being a natural effect of hitting the ball harder. Nevertheless, I *have* hit the ball harder. The ball whizzes to the baseline and the old woman can't even touch it. She looks like she has swallowed a fly. On the next point I do the same thing. She loses her serve to love. It's simple, when you think about it. I am hitting the ball harder and suddenly I am winning points. And games. Hannah does her bit too. My power combined with her accuracy works. It works well.

We win the set 6–1.

"My dinner party—" begins Hannah, looking at her watch.

"We'll just win the championship tiebreak and then you can go," I say.

I go and update the scoreboard to show we have won the set.

"Like doing it more when you're winning, don't you," says the old woman. "Your little scoreboard."

"Yes," I say. "I suppose I do."

We win the championship tiebreak.

•

I tell Dan that I'm playing in a tournament, a real one. To warm up for the Indoor Tennis Centre Open. It's in Leicester, I tell him. It's a Grade 5. He looks it up on his iPhone.

"Carpet," he says. "I love carpet."

"Is it really weird?"

"It's really fast. Like grass."

I think of the grass courts in Chelmsford. They were the exact opposite of fast.

"But it can't be that different from acrylic, though, right?"

He makes a face. "You need a game plan," he says.

•

On January 24, 2014, I watch Nadal and Federer playing in the semi-final of the Australian Open. I've never really watched much tennis before. When I was a kid, big televised tennis matches meant the courts in Central Park would be free because all the local tennis fans would be at home watching, not playing. During big tournaments was the only time you could really get a free court. I would climb up to my tree house and confirm that the courts were empty, then Couze and I would hurry through the park, hoping that the ticket inspector was also watching tennis on TV. After I abandoned tennis, I couldn't look it in the eye again for quite some time. For years, I'd simply change channels if it was on TV. Until now, actually.

It's strange to admit this, but the first time I saw Rafael Nadal play in a match was quite recently: the ATP (Association of Tennis Professionals, which governs men's professional tennis circuits) final against Djokovic in November 2013. I'd read David Foster Wallace's account of him—well, him in relation to Federer—before that, and listened to the other players in the first league match I played saying that even though Nadal was sort of attractive they wouldn't be able to bring themselves to, well, *you know*. And the first time I saw him I couldn't get over just how weird he actually was, tugging on his underwear and tucking his hair behind both ears and touching his nose before every point. I couldn't work out why people loved him so much.

Since then I've read Rafa's autobiography and his tics don't seem weird at all. In fact, I totally identify with quite a lot of his general anxiety: the fear that his mother might die if she forgets to switch off her fire at night; a terror of driving anywhere or losing control in any situation at all. The thing I never had was an Uncle Toni. If I ever did find myself as a kid watching a tennis match on TV, my mother would simply say, "You could do that. You're better than them," even if it was Martina Navratilova or John McEnroe playing. When Rafa was eight years old and forgot his bottle of water for a match, Uncle Toni made him play without water to teach him a lesson. Now, walking down the street in New York, Uncle Toni does not let Rafa walk in the middle of a group of three. "What makes you think you're so important, so special?" he apparently asks. He also usually tells Nadal he's going to lose, and that his opponent is so much better than him that if he does win it will only be because of luck.

Before I read the book, and before I really watched Nadal play, I thought I would love Federer more. And at the beginning of this match I almost think I do love Federer more, with his elegant one-handed backhand and delicate, subtle volleys. But there's Nadal at the other end, described by my new agent as a "huge piece of cow" and by David Foster Wallace as Dionysus to Federer's Apollo; war to Federer's love. Well, I have always been more of a Dionysus type of girl, but it's not just that. It's his inside-out forehand. His lasso finish. At first I don't get it, because he's left-handed and I'm not, but then I do. This is pure passion. This is beautiful. Federer might be elegant with his hair just so and his white shorts and his socks pulled up. Nadal is dirty. Gritty. Real. He has to bandage every one of his fingertips on his left hand because his extreme western grip means they will blister otherwise. Sweat pours off him all the time. This is how I want my tennis to be. Did my mother overdo the praise when

I was a kid? Undoubtedly. I look at Nadal's forehand and I want it, and I'm not going to stop until I get it, however ridiculous this is. I don't want the Nobel Prize for Literature or the FA Cup goal. I want something better. I want that forehand.

•

I am on my way down the stairs to the Indoor Tennis Centre for my 2:30 lesson with Dan. It's the last one before my very first real tournament in Leicester. I'm hoping that we'll practice the pattern of play we worked out last time, where I hit an approach shot into my opponent's backhand corner and then rush up to the net to volley away the weak return.

"Just the person I wanted to see." It's Margaret, coming down the stairs behind me. I wonder what it will be this time, how far I will have to drive or what I will have to bring, but it's not that. It's not about a match.

"Did you set your own rating on the LTA website?" she asks me.

"Yes." *Shit.* "Did I do it wrong?"

"Well, you made yourself an 8.2. That's quite high."

"Well, they gave you some choices and I said what I could do and that's what it came out as. Is there a problem?"

"Well, kind of." Margaret laughs. "You've now made yourself too high to play with Hannah in the Aegon league."

The Aegon league is the one where you can play singles. I didn't know until recently that you also have to play doubles. You go off in a team of four and play one singles and one doubles. I am haunted by doubles, which I increasingly do not like playing. But I've made a bit of a thing about the Aegon league, emailing and generally pestering Margaret about it. Ideally, I want to captain the team.

"I don't understand."

"Well, you see, in the Aegon league it's all done on ratings. As it stands, you'll be the highest. Well, I think maybe Becky's an 8.2. But Becky and Lucille have to play as the first pair and I'm not sure that'll work now."

I'm not sure why Becky and Lucille have to play as the first pair, but whatever.

"Well, I'm sorry if I've messed everything up."

We have reached the tennis center. The familiar cold, hard green of it. Dan is there with a basket of balls. It is 2:30. All I want to do is hit a ball. Show myself that I can still do it, that I will be able to do it on Sunday in Leicester. A 6.1 has just entered the tournament, which frightened me even before this conversation. If 8.2 is high, then what is 6.1 going to be like?

"I think Lucille is a 10.2," Margaret says.

"But I heard that she's an amazing player. Shouldn't she have a higher rating?"

"Well, yes, but she never plays singles, so . . ."

If she never plays singles, how does anyone know what her rating should be? But there are those descriptions on the LTA website. A 10.2 can just about keep an easy, slow rally going. A 9.2 can just about get a serve in. One of the things that made me choose 8.2 was because on this rating you can force errors with your serve. My tomahawk serve often makes people hit the ball back into the net. But of course people do get stuck with ratings that don't reflect their ability. Poor Dan has not played a tournament that affects ratings and ranking for years and is also stuck with a 9.2. If Dan is a 9.2, then the rest of us should be in the twenties. But it only goes down to 10.2, which is supposed to be for real beginners.

"I'm just not sure that my rating should change because Lucille's is wrong."

"The other problem with an 8.2 is of course that you'll end up against all the best players," Margaret points out.

Surely that's what I want? Or if not that, then at least a chance to get into better tournaments, which is the main thing a higher rating gives you. A higher rating means being closer to Wimbledon, to my agent's dream.

Margaret continues, "When I played in the Aegon league last year I just ended up being thrashed by 6.1s all the time. And then you've got county players."

Ah, the mythical county players. The stories people tell around the tennis center often involve someone accidentally playing a county player and being totally bagelled, even though no one here really calls it that. Or a county player enters a tournament that is supposed to be For Local People and thrashes everyone. I'd love to play against a county player. Especially if I could do it twice in a tournament for approximately £15. I now pay £50 a week for Dan to bagel me again and again and again. I learn an awful lot from it. Of course, what I'm really aiming for is to *be* a county player, like I almost was when I was twelve. Oh, and with a forehand like Nadal's.

"One time," Margaret says, "I was playing this county player and there I was in the corner hitting forehand after forehand and she just kept hitting them back to me and I kept hitting them back to her until then—"

"Then she smacks it down the line?"

"No, then suddenly she hits a ball about twice as fast as the others."

"Amie Tonkiss is a 7.2," I say. "And I know she was probably having an off day at the Christmas Tournament, but I did beat her."

"Yes, but that was only one set. Real matches are over three sets—"

"But I beat her 6–2. And I think I would have done the same over another set."

This is becoming weird. I was told I wouldn't beat Amie Tonkiss, and I thought I wouldn't beat her, and she beat everyone else in that tournament except me, but I did beat her. I won. But now it's as if that was some kind of freak result and because I shouldn't have beaten her on some level, I didn't. It's as if it doesn't count.

Actually, every person I have played at singles in this tennis center, in this vast green rectangle, *every single one* apart from the Level 3 coaches, I have beaten. I beat everyone I played in the Christmas Tournament. On club nights I have beaten Cheryl 6–2, Tim 6–1, Lee 6–0, Carolla 6–0. I played a couple of sets with Cheryl just after Christmas, 6–2, 6–1. I am not so conceited that I am not totally surprised every time this happens. And I am not such an idiot that I think I'm going to go out there and have the same sorts of results against 6.1s, or even other 8.2s, or all the 10.2s and 9.2s out there who are hiding their ability behind the wrong numbers, like two-bottles-of-wine Gemma (a 10.2 apparently) and the mysterious Lucille. I have been prepared, for weeks now, to go to Leicester and get quadruple-bagelled over my two matches. I have yet to take a game off Dan. But I have had him at deuce a couple of times recently, and once at 30–0. Hayley Palmer, Dan's official doubles partner, for whom I seem now to be the regular reserve, is an 8.2. Hayley and Becky (also an 8.2) would both give me a good game at singles, I know that. I am actually terrified of the day I end up playing Hayley, because I think she might 7–5 me. But I don't think she could bagel me. Same with Becky, although I feel more terrified of playing Becky.

"Most people," Margaret says, "start at 10.2 or 9.2 and work their way up."

"Look, I am sorry," I say. "Really. But the LTA site just said to be as honest as possible about your abilities and the descriptions of 10.2 and 9.2 just didn't seem to match up. But I really am sorry if I've messed everything up. Honestly, if you think it would be best to just leave me out of the Aegon team then I really don't mind."

"No! Don't be silly."

I begin my coaching session ten minutes late. Am I really that much worse than I think I am? Have I so overestimated my abilities that I just come across as deluded and ridiculous? But I have a trophy! I was in the local paper! Even though people didn't think I could have beaten Amie or that I should have beaten Amie, I did beat her. I did. *But only over one set*, says Margaret's voice in my head. *Real matches are . . .* Fuck. Is this what it's going to be like during my tournament? Every time I think I can do it, will Margaret's voice materialize in my head and tell me I can't? I whack the ball really hard to Dan, tears forming in my eyes. *I'm not that bad!* We keep hard-hitting rallies going for ten or twenty shots and the mistakes that end them are not all mine. This time I take Dan to advantage in one game, and 40–30 in another. But I still have not won a game off him. Not that I really expect to—or, on some level, really want to.

2

Leicester

It's February 1, 2014. I'm at St. Pancras station and I can't settle. I almost had a panic attack in a tunnel on the train here, which hasn't happened for a long time. I have an hour to wait for my train to Leicester, and I'm carrying too much stuff. I am terrified of one of those stupid injuries one gets from simply lifting a bag onto a train or lugging things up or down stairs. I go to Foyles and buy a book on mindfulness. My wheeled bag keeps bashing me, or maybe I keep walking into it. I have that incredible lack of coordination I remember from job interviews and first dates. I basically have the Elbow and I'm not even in Leicestershire. I can't put my number into an ATM properly. I can't put my bag on a chair at Patisserie Valerie. My breathing is shallow and pathetic. I order a peppermint tea I don't even want just to take up another few minutes and then I burn my tongue with it. Then I give myself twenty minutes to make the four-minute journey from where I am sitting to Platform 4.

Once I am on the train, I start worrying about getting off. What if the door doesn't open? What if I leave my racquets behind? I used to just stick them in my big Adidas bag along with my other stuff, but now I have a special red Wilson two-racquet bag that I'm very fond of but unused to carrying around with me. I am so worried about leaving it behind on the train that I end up sitting with it on my lap. I am not sure what I have turned into. I'm pretty sure that until recently I was quite cool and didn't worry about things like this. I'm the kind of person who leaves my iPad behind on the table when I go to the toilet on a train on the basis that no one would be daring enough to actually steal it and if they did I could just get a new one.

But competitive tennis throws up all sorts of problems for which there may be no solution. Run out of moisturizer while traveling? There are thousands of places to buy moisturizer. But break a shoe-lace or lose your tennis racquets? You are fucked, my friend. My tennis shoes are bright green Asics Gel Speeds that you can't get in very many places, and every other type of trainer gives me blisters or breaks my toes or slows me down in some other way. I also do rather like the color. If something went wrong with one of them I would just cry. This is why I have two identical pairs and they are both in my suitcase, which is also why I really mustn't leave my suitcase behind.

At Leicester station I get the lift up to the exit—because I have so much stuff, and because of my knees—and end up in an odd deserted tunnel with ticket barriers that won't let me out no matter how many times I put my ticket through them. I swear at them. I kick them. I think how stupid it would be if I injured myself kicking ticket barriers at Leicester station. A uniformed bloke appears but when I ask him for help, he tells me I have to press the help button behind me. I do this and when I'm asked what the problem is I say the problem is that these stupid gates won't let me out. There is a long pause. "*Stupid* are they?" comes a superior male voice. I have lost my cool, and time, efficiency, face. Basically, I'm a fucking idiot. Eventually they let me out and I shuffle off quietly and get in a cab.

The Hilton is nice. Maybe David's right and I would have got more mileage out of a Travelodge. Still, here it is, off the M2 between Sainsbury's and Pets at Home, and even though it is nice I wonder why anyone would stay here if they didn't have a tennis tournament ten minutes down the road. Anyway, I'm here now and I do have a tennis match. Tomorrow. 3:00 p.m. I almost can't breathe.

When I check in, I ask about the spa and whether it's normal to just go there in your dressing gown.

"Sorry, Ms. Thomas, but you don't have a dressing gown as part of your package."

"Oh dear."

"You have a complimentary snack basket."

"I think I'd prefer a dressing gown."

"OK, that's all right. We can easily send one to you. That's not a problem."

"Great. I mean I'd definitely rather have that." I laugh. "I'll swap my snack basket for a dressing gown if you like."

She laughs too.

"Is there anything else I can help you with, Ms. Thomas?"

I book a table for dinner. A taxi for tomorrow.

When I get to my room there is no basket, but there is a jar of nuts next to two small bottles of mineral water. I have to chase the dressing gown, but eventually a young guy turns up with one in a plastic wrapper. But he does not give it to me immediately; he just stands there holding it. What on earth?

"She said you had something to give me in return," he says, almost in a whisper.

"Sorry?"

"Like you were swapping it for something?" he looks up and down the corridor. What kind of transaction is this exactly? Then I realize.

"Oh, I see. My, er—" It seems inappropriate to call a jar of nuts a snack basket. "My, er, *nuts*. Right. Well. I mean, I was only joking around really, but do take them." I go and get them off the desk.

He realizes what's happened. "Oh no," he says, laughing. "You're all right."

"Really, take them. I won't eat them."

"No, you're all right. You keep them."

He leaves without the nuts.

This definitely would not happen in a Travelodge.

•

The Leicester Hilton. I go for a drink in the bar. France is playing England in the Six Nations rugby championship. There are a few families here, a small handful of lone men. It's the weekend, so there are fewer business travelers than I guess there would usually be. On closer inspection, one of the families is actually a date. The kid sits there with headphones on while Mum and her new bloke swap stories of their childhoods. When France scores the winning try against England, she says her birthday is now ruined. When the kid takes off his headphones, the man tells him that the orange juice he just drank will actively rot his teeth for the next twenty minutes.

I think of Rod at home watching this rugby game and wonder again why I am here. I order another glass of wine, which I take through to the almost empty dining room, where I watch Nadal hit forehand after forehand on my iPad while I eat overcooked steak and oven chips. I wonder how difficult it is to win a tennis tournament. I wonder when it will happen to me and whether it might be tomorrow. It does not occur to me that it might never happen: that

I might never win another tennis tournament, that the Christmas tournament was just a strange random blip in my life.

Before I go to sleep, I write a plan on my iPhone that I can follow tomorrow when I am too nervous to work out what to do next.

Get up—8:45

Breakfast—9:00/9:15

Breathing and meditation—10:00

Go to swimming pool and relax—10:45

Arrive back from swimming and have shower—11:30

Lunch—12:00 check all-day menu available in bar

Get ready—1:00

Leave in cab—1:45

First match—3:00

On the way to breakfast on Sunday morning I go to the front desk to make sure my taxi is booked for 1:45. The tennis center is apparently no more than fifteen minutes away, although sometimes there is traffic. My first match is at 3:00. I had originally booked a taxi for 12:45, but realized last night this was too early even for me and so, after my lonely dinner with Nadal's digital ghost, I went to the desk to change the time. I am accustomed to waiting an hour for things. In fact, because I am always an hour early for anything important, I kind of know what to do with that hour. A couple of pees. Lipstick. A bit of reading. Instagram, perhaps. But two hours? It's too much.

Anyway, checking at the desk should just be a formality. I definitely changed the booking last night. All I want is a *Yes, Ms. Thomas. That's all been booked for you.*

"Who did you speak to?" asks Zara at the desk.

"Um, I don't remember."

She sighs. "It's just we book taxis with two companies. Do you know which one she called?"

It's early and I haven't had breakfast.

"No one told me when I made the booking that I would have to memorize both the name of the person who made it and who she made it with."

I am Ollie from *The Seed Collectors*. Bryony, even.

She rings both firms. Neither has my booking. She makes the booking.

Of course, at 1:45 two taxis will turn up.

And just before that I will get a text saying *Sorry no coaches Dave.*

•

Everything in Leicester smells of Lynx men's deodorant. I have done my breathing and meditation and now it's time to go to the pool to relax, as per my plan. But it's hard to relax when everything smells of Lynx. There's something going on in the swimming pool called Splash Time—children, brightly colored plastic, noise, pee in the pool—so I go and hide in the sauna. I am going to meditate, to keep chipping away at the ego that is holding me back not just from spiritual perfection but also from the gritty, earthly business of winning tennis matches. I'm not sure the two aims are at all compatible, but never mind.

There are two young guys in the sauna already.

"Legs," one is saying to the other. "I just don't see the point in legs."

"Greg loves legs."

"Yeah, right? But I can't see the point in it. Abs, chest, and biceps, that's all anyone cares about. Not fucking legs."

"No."

"I mean who even sees your legs? I don't think anyone's ever looked at my calves. And fucking shoulders? You might as well exercise your ears."

•

I am trying to do something about my ego. This has been going on for a while now. A couple of years ago a therapist introduced me to *A Course in Miracles*. Did I think I'd become the type of person who would spend fifty minutes every Tuesday afternoon in a suburban sitting room with scented candles, talking about my childhood and trying to become perfect inside as well as out? When did I become that, rather than the cool, chain-smoking linguist with flats in Paris and Rome that my fifteen-year-old self would have wanted to be? But when the therapist says mysterious things like "You are loved, whatever you do" and "You are perfect just as you are," something deep inside of me takes notice. These are messages I'm not hearing anywhere else. I'm not even really hearing them from her, either; what I'm hearing is that I should begin a lengthy program to get rid of the ego that tells me I am better and different so that I can be better and different. My life becomes a paradox, but at least it's interesting. Instead of moaning about my childhood, I am to forgive everyone. Life does become easier when I do this, although I usually forget.

•

The David Lloyd Tennis Centre Narborough, known locally as simply "the health club" according to my cab driver—who, when I ask him to slow down, simply grasps my arm, cackles, and says, "You all right baby, innit?"—is stuck down at the wrong end of a lonely industrial estate alongside warehouses and huge buildings that appear to have no windows. Some buildings have recognizable names on them, but there are no people. It's like L.A. would be after a mild nuclear disaster.

"You are tennis player, baby? Professional?"

When cab drivers ask what I do, there usually follows an awkward conversation about whether I have ever had anything published and if it falls into the category of "romance" or "crime." This is new. Of course, at this moment I look nothing like a professional. My skirt and top are both black Adidas, but I am still modeling my look on the best players at the Indoor Tennis Centre, not, as I will do later, the prettiest players on the WTA Tour who have "pro collections" on Tennisnuts.co.uk.

"Ha ha," I say. "I wish!"

Sometimes I turn up to do a reading at a bookshop and there's that moment when I arrive and the shop is officially closed and so someone says something like, "Can I help you?" or "Do you have a ticket?" and I smile and say "Actually I'm Scarlett Thomas," and there's a bit of embarrassment and fluster and I'm shown upstairs to the staff room or passed over to someone who does recognize me and sometimes even seems excited to meet me and I feel special and kind of at peace.

Here, at the David Lloyd Tennis Centre Narborough, there are gray turnstiles I'm not even sure I'm going to be allowed through. I do not belong here. I am not a member. I don't know where I am. I don't know what is beyond the turnstiles. I am a mess of anxiety. It's just like on the train. For example, I *know* I have my purse and my phone with me, but what if I'd actually left them in the cab? What if I was stuck here on this lonely industrial estate without the two things that give me the only safety and power I have in this world? Or—perhaps worse—what if I'd left my tennis racquets behind and it is now 2:59 and a man is looking at his watch and saying "If you can't find a new racquet in one minute we'll have to disqualify you"? But I have my money and my phone and my racquets. All is well. But I do not feel calm. I still feel as if I am in the nightmare version of this. What if it's been canceled? Moved? What if someone thinks I'm not eligible to play for some reason? In the nightmare version of this, someone would probably hand me a horse and tell me I had to walk around the building with it fifteen times before play commences in five minutes. What if they just don't let me through the turnstiles?

They do. But they also tell me that if I leave I won't be able to get back in again. Presumably they don't mean it. But I hate these stupid situations where you have to negotiate every time you want to do something.

"The tennis people are over there," they say, pointing toward the bar.

"And is it possible for me to use the gym beforehand, to warm up?"

"Not without membership."

"Right."

Oh God. I shouldn't have come. This is fucking stupid. What am I doing here in Leicestershire, in the middle of nowhere, in a place where I can't use the gym or book a coach to help me get used to the surface before I play on it? This was supposed to be me living out my fantasy of being a tennis star. Instead it's . . . I don't know. As I walk over to the bar area, I see a guy of about my age who is a little bit too fat for the tennis outfit he is wearing. He has a preposterous headband. Is he a local character? He goes onto court to begin his singles match against a dumpy man with glasses. All his shots are weird. I begin to think disparaging thoughts about how old and embarrassing everyone looks and then realize that I must look exactly the same. I'd thought a tennis tournament might be glamorous. I'd imagined a shining sports venue with tiered seating and young, toned competitors stretching and chatting. But this is to Wimbledon what a sales conference disco is to the Royal Ballet. We are all fooling ourselves. I find a guy with a clipboard and tell him my name. He ticks it off without even looking at me. "You're on at 3:00 p.m.," he says. "Your opponent isn't here yet." I thank him and sit down at one of the round tables with a view of what I will later learn are called "show courts." I get a cup of tea from the bar, mainly as something to do. I shouldn't drink too much tea: it makes me pee, and I'm certain that the caffeine has been making me jittery lately. Still, if it's good enough for Kenyan runners . . .

Then a vision appears. She is thin, tall, and dressed in an Adidas tennis outfit I recognize from the Australian Open. She is carrying the biggest tennis bag I have ever seen. I thought I was a bit stuck-up with my two racquets in a matching bag, but this woman's bag is like something off the TV. It is red and silver: the latest Wilson bag, designed to carry at least six racquets and a change of clothes. I am terrified just looking at her. She must be an awesome player to have a bag that big. If I put my stuff in a bag that big everyone would just laugh at me, right? At last, though, some glamour. Is she my opponent? I really hope not. There's a Black girl with a crew cut warming up on Court 2. She has a guy with her; he's feeding her balls and she's swatting them back like something from *Tomb Raider*. Maybe I'd even rather play her than this professional-looking woman who has just arrived. But no, she is put on to play against a slim Asian-looking girl who looks even more nervous than me.

The glamorous woman is put on to play against a sturdy-looking Black girl with glasses and wild, impressive hair. The glamorous woman's good-looking boyfriend pulls a chair as close as possible to the glass screen to watch her. I wish Rod were here to watch me. I ache for some love, some reassurance, someone to care about my performance. Everyone else here seems to have someone. Most of all, at this moment, I want a gang. It has become clear that the girl with the crew cut and the girl with the wild hair have arrived together. Also in their entourage: several cool guys and a well-built Spanish-looking woman with long dark hair and a blue Nike T-shirt over some sloppy shorts. This must be Natalia Lozano, my opponent. I have been stalking all the players on the LTA website and I remember that Natalia was the one with the 7.2 rating but no actual matches played, which means she gave the rating to herself. Which might mean—I hope it means—that she is really shit but quite up-herself.

On Court 1, the woman with the huge bag is about to serve. She throws the ball up—not very high, I note—and then something bizarre happens. After a flurry of racquet and a blur of green, the ball is rolling awkwardly on the ground in front of her and her left fist is all scrunched up and her knees sort of buckle and she looks as if she might cry. She is so nervous that she has not hit the ball. Her second serve goes into the net. Her hands are shaking. She curses herself, quietly. The boyfriend is on the edge of his seat, visibly willing her on. She glances at him from time to time, looking unhappy and still on the verge of tears. Soon it becomes too embarrassing to watch. She can barely hit the ball, and her opponent—who also seems to fluff a lot of shots, not that it matters—beats her 6–0, 6–1. The one game the woman gets is due to four double faults from her opponent. But this is all very interesting. It turns out you can have a great outfit and a huge bag and actually be extremely shit. I file this information away to think about properly later. I wish I had been playing her. If I had been playing her, I would now be through to the second round of my first-ever tournament.

Brad Gilbert is going around my head like something at a Grand Prix. All his neat examples of the things you can do to prepare for your match are scrambling in my mind. The guy who, before a match, arrives at the venue and secretly hits with a coach before having a stretch and a shower and appearing, ready for his match (with a final twist, which Brad disapproves of, where he deliberately arrives late and suggests going straight into the match with no warm-up). I would do that except there is no coach, and no showers. I'm tired. My muscles feel stiff. I've spent the day building up to this, but none of my preparations have come to much. I'm not even warm. At this moment, when I am surely due to go on any minute, *I am not even warm*. Not even slightly. For fuck's sake. I go downstairs for a pee. The loos are next to the gym. There is nothing stopping anyone from going to the gym. I get my bag and go to the gym. My stomach churns, nervous with acid.

My current playlist is full of stuff from the *Girls* soundtrack. There's a Rolling Stones song, "Fool to Cry," that I listened to all the time when I was going through my Stones phase when I was sixteen or seventeen. Listening to it now, I wonder why on earth I was obsessed with something so sad, so, well, *taboo*. It's about a kid comforting her father. I tend to avoid things to do with fathers, especially girls and their fathers. Sad fathers. Missing fathers. Anxious fathers. Then I realize that all those years ago I thought the lyric was about someone named Danny, not Daddy, and that's why I liked the song. Guess I missed the bit where the protagonist puts daughter on his knee, the bit I hear so clearly now through my Bluetooth headphones, and she says, "Daddy, you're a fool to cry . . ."

The day they told me that Gordian was my father is kind of a blur. In some versions, Steve has not yet left for America; in others, it's *because* he's left that they think it's the right time to tell me, as if fathers worked a bit like revolving doors: one out, one in. I'm twelve. It happens in Chelmsford, in the study filled with books about Freud and post-structuralist theory. Perhaps we've already played tennis that morning, or will later. I play tennis with Couze all the time, of course, but playing with Gordian is a special weekend treat. Sometimes Couze and Gordian will play together; occasionally my mother plays too, all giggly and unrealistically competitive. I always feel left out of their adult world, with its incomprehensible dynamics.

Given this, I might even be wearing my favorite tennis outfit: a pleated white skirt with a little metal clasp, a matching white polo top, and matching white sweatbands for my wrists and forehead. Couze will know that something big is happening, and he will be doing something supportive in the kitchen: tea for everyone, or prepping the Sunday roast.

I'm probably sitting on the faded red beanbag. Mum and Gordian are on antique chairs, brimming with secrecy. There's something credulous and naïve about me. Mum says, "There's something we want to tell you." Dramatic pause. "Steve isn't your father." And here's where I'm a bit stupid, or maybe it's the screenwriter in me coming out early. "Who is?" I say, not really doing the math; not really thinking about who's in the room. And so Gordian gets to say his line, the one he must have been rehearsing in some way for the last twelve years.

"I am."

Afterward, walking up the stairs to my bedroom, I recall finding myself frustratingly unchanged. I wanted to feel like a fairy-tale princess, or like a character from the YA books I read, but instead I was experiencing something that still happens to me when I get good news (and at the time, this was very good news, because Steve was weird and wore black clothes and could be a bit violent, while Gordian was kind and exotic and brought me expensive presents). I felt a bit flat, slightly crushed, anticlimactic. The now-familiar thought: *Can I live up to this, or will I let everyone down somehow?* And *How do I become the perfect daughter of* this *man, rather than the other one?* Steve wanted me to like computers and video games and punky, counterculture things. He took me to Hells Angels parties where I once even got to (and let's not think about this too much) kiss a musician named Buster Bloodvessel. And of course there's Couze, who wanted me to be sporty and intellectual and understand French and philosophy. What will this third father want from me?

Now, in Leicester, I flick my playlist forward and listen to Sugarman instead. My legs go round and round on the elliptical as I try to get warm without getting too tired but fail. I am so nervous. I wish this would end. I wish it would begin. I go back upstairs and then almost immediately have to come back down for another pee.

Finally, at around 3:45, I am given a tube of three—only three!—balls and told to go to Court 3. We're to play "short sets." WTF? The guy with the clipboard explains that this means the sets are to four games rather than six, clear by two games, with a tiebreak on 5–5, if it comes to that. Oh no! So I have come all this way and paid all this money and got a hotel and now we're playing short bloody sets with only three balls. I try to act as professional and confident as possible, although I have no real idea what this means any more. I have three bottles of drink: electrolyte water, plain water, and Coke. I take them out and put them where I can easily reach them on changeovers, but really, I want to cry. Natalia starts chatting about her job in London and how she's just got back into tennis after playing as a kid and this is her first tournament. Remembering all Brad's advice, I say nothing. I let Natalia lead the warm-up. I can only vaguely remember how you do it. In Brad's world this means I have already lost, but there's nothing else I can do. The ball bounces strangely on the carpet. Natalia hits it hard, early, with a lot of topspin. When I accidentally lob her, she hotdogs the ball back. This is so incredibly cool, or would be if I weren't about to play her. A hotdog! Dan occasionally does these; Josh does them all the time. It's where you've run to the baseline for a ball but don't have time to turn around, so you hit the ball back between your legs. Federer hits winners like this. I have never seen a girl do one.

Dan's best shot is a killer forehand that he times perfectly and—*thwack!*—the ball is so fast it is unplayable, wherever it lands on the court. He does this shot sometimes in coaching or in the Reccy sessions, to indicate he's bored, or just to show off, and it's the coolest thing I have ever seen. To stop him doing it against me when we play for points, I have to keep the ball deep. Later I will learn how to play to his backhand and eliminate the shot altogether—although by then I will often be able to get it back. But this is the forehand I want. This is the forehand for which, if I met some shady character in a dark forest late at night who offered it to me for some price, I would pay that price, any price. I would almost—will almost, but we'll come to that—die for this forehand. Just to hit it once. Natalia has this forehand. She hits it a few times in the warm-up.

She wins the toss, decides to serve (Brad says you should always receive, of course, and so I think this means she is tactically inept, which surely means I am in with a chance?). Her first serve: an ace. Her next one: an ace. It's 30–0. Next serve in the net. Joy! Next serve: an ace. I manage to return her serve on 40–0. It's a pathetic backhand down the line, but at least I have hit the ball. She does the forehand of doom right back at me. There's so much top-spin on it, and the carpet plays so fast, that the ball only bounces once before thwacking hard into the heavy curtain behind me. By the time I even try to play the ball, it is long gone. Oh lord. But it's OK! Brad says that everyone is beatable: you just have to work out how to beat them. Natalia will have a weakness; I just need to find out what it is.

Now I am to serve. I plonk it in the box and—*thwack!*—it's that forehand again, down the line on my backhand side, quick bounce and then straight into the curtain. I serve to her ad side and it's the same again, although this time the forehand is crosscourt and it hits the netting separating us from Court 2. It's the same again for the next two points, and the first set is over in a blur. I think I win maybe one more point when she hits the ball out. She takes the first set 4–0. Oh dear.

Natalia serves like Dan. In fact, she does everything a bit like Dan. She serves according to where you stand. I have only read about this in books and seen it on TV, but it actually exists. I told myself I could not possibly meet someone as good as Dan in a tournament like this, but here she is. In the second set I concentrate as hard as I can. My serve is working, although it feels like a huge effort of strength and concentration. But all my safe hesitant shots are simply blasted down my backhand side behind me. I know that the only way I will win is if she dies or breaks her leg before the end. But I somehow take two games off her.

She has a grunt, too. Natalia's grunt is professional and amazing. It sounds like "lick-air." A couple of times I think she's calling my serve long, but she's just exhaling loudly as she returns it. Lick-air. Indeed. It's what her forehand does.

•

It's dark and cold and I'm into the consolation draw. My next opponent is Charanya Ravi, 9.1. She is a sweet, slightly frail-looking student who apologizes during the warm-up that she's rubbish at feeding volleys. She has just been double-bagelled by the crew-cut girl, Meredith. We really need the warm-up. We have been sent outside onto a court that is, improbably, just more carpet but a kind of outdoor green version. A worm is dying in the deuce court service box. I want to help it, but I can't. There is no real earth here. When I run for a backhand I slip and almost do the splits. In a bad way, not at all like Djokovic. This crunchy stuff? Yes, it's frost. I am playing on frozen Astroturf. I wear several layers, leg warmers, and my woolly hat. Charanya wears all of this and gloves. I can't remember what any of my tennis books say about wind, but there is some. It means that in the first game Charanya's first serve sort of stops in the service box and then goes backward. The balls become soggy, then fluffy. I wonder if eventually they too will freeze.

She's not a bad player, but somehow I win 4–2, 4–1. I only got up to the net against Natalia once, but with Charanya I manage it a good handful of times. I even win three or four points from my planned pattern. This match is slower (and colder and windier), but it also goes past in a bit of a blur. There are not many long rallies. I am sure that if I move too fast I am going to slip and fall, but I never feel like I really hit out or lose myself in a point. I am painfully aware of the score at all times. I rescue several break points. I am tenacious. I am freezing cold. I am also ignoring Brad and chatting. I find out that Charanya is a student at Oxford, although I don't ask what she's studying. She says she's surprised that this tournament even went ahead. Apparently they don't usually get enough entrants to run the ladies' singles events in Grade 5s. *People drop out at the last minute,* Charanya says. *They do it all the time.*

I'm in the consolation draw final! I have a cup of tea and warm up inside, but Kevin Clipboard seems to think we should play outside again. It is now 6:00 p.m. and we are in the East Midlands on February 2. I begin nicely, almost a tiny bit flirtatiously. "Please, please don't make us play outside again. It's so cold and dark and icy." When this fails to move him, I add darkly, "and dangerous." He says he'll try to find us an indoor court, but unfortunately the tournament organizer has accidentally only booked the courts until 6:00 p.m., not 8:00 p.m. People are turning up for their evening hit about. Natalia is playing Crystal (6.1) on Court 2 in the ladies' final. But we can't have that next because Kevin wants to put the men's final on it. He walks around with his clipboard for a while. Rings Simon, the tournament organizer. Talks to a David Lloyd person.

"Right," he says. "According to Simon you don't actually have to play the consolation draw final. You're only guaranteed two matches. We don't have to give you a third one. So unless you want to play outside . . ."

We agree to play outside. But once Sally, my opponent, has gone to get changed, I have a bright idea. I ask Kevin if anyone would be willing to give us their court for £20. Perhaps sensing how desperate I really am not to go outside, he magically finds us a court. It's been booked from 6:00, but the people haven't shown up. It is booked again at 7:00. It is now 6:10. If the people who have booked it show up, then they are within their rights to kick us off the court.

I am furious—pleased of course that I don't have to go outside again, but furious that I have paid my match fee and traveled here and got a hotel and basically done my bit only to be faced with lackluster organization and a sense that what I have come here to do does not matter to anyone. In order to have any chance of playing singles seriously, I have had to travel to Leicester. But what I was looking for isn't here. I should have pulled out when I was unable to get a hit on the surface beforehand.

I'm not yet totally crushed, but it is not my best self that goes into the final with Sally Foster, 8.2. I am particularly anxious about being thrown off the court. And I never do well when I am being treated badly. I tend to step up when there is glamour, pizazz, any kind of audience and excitement and pressure. Here on Court 5, away from the show courts, the only people around are a dad teaching his son to grunt while playing his badminton shots. "Just like a tennis player," he says. But I am not grunting. Grunting is on my list of things I must do but I am not doing it.

But I do enjoy my match against Sally. She is a pusher—someone who plays steadily and waits for you to make a mistake—and a good one, which means at least we can have long rallies. We are both nervous, and have both lost some concentration. Afterward, she admits to shaking with nerves. I'm not doing that any more. I can serve without stage fright and everything. But I am still—still—not hitting out. I am not finishing my shots. I am not grunting. I am hitting the ball middle and deep and she is standing in the middle and I am standing in the middle and we middle-and-deep the ball back to each other and could this be the first time I have been *bored* playing tennis? A few moonballs. I try to work my way up to the net a few times. I win a few points this way, but she passes me a couple of times and lobs me.

Sally is a confident, tight player. And I do enjoy those rallies, when I am not glancing at the door to see if we are about to lose our court. She wins her first service game and then I win mine and then she breaks me and wins the set 4–1. I serve a couple of double faults.

I am tired, not so much physically but mentally. I start serving flat because I can't be bothered to change my grip for my spin serve. Still, I do get it where I want to a lot of the time, including out to the backhand on the ad side, which is a new serve for me. But Sally gets them all back.

At 7:00 p.m. it is 3–2 in the second set. I am trying to gear myself up to win the next three games and take this to a championship tiebreak when Kevin comes in with his clipboard. He wants to know the score. When I tell him, he looks pleased. We'll surely only be a few minutes while Sally takes this final game. I have struggled to get any focus at all today, and the small amount of concentration I had left is now gone. To her credit, Sally serves like she really wants this win. And I do try to take the game, I really do. Sort of. But by now I also sort of want to go home.

Afterward Sally says she has enjoyed this match most in the day. And indeed, we have been able to play boring, polite white-girl tennis and not had to compete with frighteningly cool Black girls or sassy Spaniards from London. I hate myself. As much as I like and respect Sally, I so, so desperately want to play tennis like the other girls. I want to be in their gang. I'd literally give anything.

•

I have not had money long enough to have learned that you can't simply buy anything you want or need. Despite my refined genes, I spent the first part of my life in a council flat in Barking before we eventually moved to Chelmsford to live with Couze when I was nine. Sometimes people ask me what I enjoyed most in my early childhood. Well, I really, really loved my mum. I liked toast, and Enid Blyton's Faraway Tree books. Otherwise, there was nothing.

I watched my little dog Rags get run over when I was eight. School was a confusing world of shame. Boys laughed at everything I did. Everyone was racist, sexist, poor. Everyone smoked, and it was common for people to simply use their carpet as an ashtray. You just flick the ash on it and rub it in with your foot. That's what all the adults around me did. I played in a dump. Worried about going to hell. Tried to forget the inappropriate horror stories the cackly ladies on the estate told me about rats eating pregnant women's stomachs (a battered James Herbert book had been doing the rounds). The man in the flat below us had bed bugs. My grandmother died. My grandfather had his leg amputated and then died. And then later, of course, I discovered that they'd never even been my grandparents.

After Rags died I didn't wash the blood off my arm for days. Rags had been my best friend; I couldn't get over his death. My mother didn't know what to do with me, so she sent me to Gordian. I didn't yet know he was my father. He was in the Manor Recording studio in Oxfordshire with the band he managed, OMD, who were recording their new album. I stayed there with them for two weeks, messing around in the pool with the band, eating real adult food, learning to cross my 7s like sophisticated people did, feeling that *this* was how my life should be. But any time I caught myself feeling happy, even for a second, an image of the white van hitting Rags would fill my mind. His little body lying in the gutter.

Even now it makes me want to cry.

The first chunk of money I ever got was a slightly dodgy insurance claim after Mum and I were in a minor car accident when I was twenty-one. It was a few hundred quid and I spent it paying off debts and buying a Stüssy hoodie. When my novel *The End of Mr. Y* became a surprise success in 2007, I bought shoes: leather ballerinas, which made me feel guilty because I'd been a vegan for ages. They cost £69.99 and came from Russell and Bromley. I'd never spent more than about £25 on shoes before. When I was a kid, Gordian had money, and Mum thought he could use it to solve anything. If ever I wanted or needed anything expensive, I'd have to phone him and ask him for it. He paid for my two tennis holidays, and my tennis racquets.

By the time I was sixteen, I'd gone from real poverty in Barking with Steve to a comfortable but not very flush suburban boho existence with Couze, which involved reading the *Guardian*, making marmalade, and saving string. But always there were these random flashes of Gordian, the rich, glamorous, Jewish superhero, suddenly taking us all for expensive restaurant lunches and even employing, in his bachelor flat in Islington, a *cleaner*. It was fashionable in the 1980s for bands to own part-shares in a racehorse, and so I had a few fun times at the racetrack with Gordian, where I was allowed to gamble and keep my winnings, and I learned to drink cocktails (always a Virgin Mary back then, with extra Tabasco and a stick of celery) and ask about chart positions and what they meant.

Today in Leicester I'm beginning to understand all the things money can't buy. I couldn't get a warm-up hit with a coach here even though I was willing to pay. I couldn't buy my way onto a tennis court for my ridiculous "final" with Sally. And of course now, at the end of rather a disillusioning day, I cannot buy mobile phone reception when there is none. I can't leave this place because I won't be able to get back in, but I also can't get any signal on my phone. It is dark and cold. Natalia, Meredith, and the others are sitting around a table together laughing and chatting. I don't want them to see me crying. I find a tiny pocket of mobile phone reception—two bars? No, just one—by the door to the toilet but there's no way I can get any data, so I can't look up cab numbers. I have to ask behind the bar. But they don't know any cab numbers so I have to ask at reception. Brad Gilbert certainly never covered what to do in this scenario where you are a total loser stuck in a room with a bunch of winners and you need to leave but can't.

Eventually I get through to a cab company. But it can't send a cab for at least another two hours. Two fucking hours! What kind of place is this? I want to storm around proclaiming everyone to be enormous *cunts* and everything to be a fucking pile of ginormous *shit* but I don't have enough self-esteem left to do this, even in my imagination. Really, I just want to cry quietly on my own somewhere. I have to get out of here. What can I realistically do? I would book a helicopter if I could. Offer my firstborn to a goblin who would ... Hang on. Didn't the cab driver who brought me here give me a receipt? And might the receipt have their number on it? I fish around in my bag. *Yes.* It's a Leicester cab company rather than a Narborough one. I call them. They can have a cab here in half an hour.

•

The moon is crisp and white: a thin nail clipping from a big thumbs-down. This time the cab driver does not ask me if I am a professional tennis player.

Oh, how we delude ourselves with sport. I watch Serena and Azarenka on TV and I think that what I am watching is what I do. I still can't convince myself that with enough effort I can't do that. What is wrong with me? This has been a big mistake.

Back at the Hilton and I am hungry, exhausted, tearful. My legs hurt, a lot. On the other hand—I got to a final! OK, it was only the consolation draw final, but still. I beat Charanya. I mean, this was my first-ever tournament and I beat someone! I order a glass of white wine and some dinner and phone Rod.

I speak to Rod for ages, telling him everything that happened. Then my mother rings and I tell her the same story but I feel a bit silly. I'm a middle-aged woman talking to my mother about my first tennis tournament. Of course, she can't understand why I haven't won it. Then I do it all over again with Couze, who is impressed, and sweet, and says maybe he should take up tennis and we can play again, like we used to. He's supposed to be exercising more, after all.

The Hilton is doing my head in. Anything that does not run away gets put in the deep fryer. My pan-fried potato and spinach cake has not been in a pan. It has been in a basket and lowered into bubbling brown vegetable oil. Even my new potato mash may have been in the deep fryer for a few moments. I have started thinking that if you can deep-fry an egg (which is what they do at breakfast) you can deep-fry anything, and it's giving me the willies. I am even a little suspicious of my chocolate ice cream. Could you deep-fry something and then freeze it? Isn't that basically how they make all junk food in this country anyway? I order another £8.50 glass of wine to take back to my room but then tip half of it down the sink because I'm worried about drinking too much.

On the way home, I watch too-wet landscapes flood past while the East Midland Trains cups clink against one another on the First Class table. I feel changed, somehow, like when I finally lost my virginity to beautiful, curly-haired Justin, when I was sixteen. I've done it. *I've done it.* I've played my first ever tennis tournament. On Monday, back in my office, I take a break from my admin blitz and google the mysterious Natalia Lozano. Turns out she was in the top twenty in Spain as a junior and reached number 59 nationally as a senior. So maybe taking two games off her was quite good.

•

One of the main things I have learned since having a moderate amount of success and making some money: normal life is on hold as long as you are in a hotel room. Anything you eat or drink in a hotel room does not count. Anything you feel in a hotel room does not count. This must be why people have affairs in hotel rooms. As long as you are traveling, you don't have to face life. As long as you have some train tickets in your purse and an email from Laterooms.com, then everything is OK. You can run and life can't catch you. The concept of the tennis tournament is an extension of this. I am signed up for something. I am in a draw. As long as my name is written on a piece of paper somewhere, there is proof that I exist. So while the Leicester experience should have put me off, it has not. In fact, I immediately begin looking for more tournaments I can enter. I don't care where they are.

3

Ragdale Hall

I am sitting in a redbrick building in the East Midlands refreshing the LTA "Player" page over and over again. *Fault*, it keeps saying. *Sorry.* The latest ratings run is due and I know that once it is complete I will, for the very first time ever, have a national and county ranking for tennis. I know my rating will not change this time. I have not even beaten one person with a higher rating than me, let alone the three required, so I will remain an 8.2. But I have some ranking points for reaching the final of the consolation draw of the David Lloyd Narborough Way2Play tournament last week. Twenty, to be precise. What does twenty ranking points get you? It's the kind of thing my mother gets impossibly excited about. Will I now be number 1 in the county? Unlikely. The country? *Mother!* Mum is here, in her superior double room next door, but I won't tell her I am doing this. I will keep secretly refreshing the page until I have confirmation of the place I now am. Somewhere to say, *This is where I am now*, and then, *That is where I am going.* But not to anyone else. Not yet.

I am at Ragdale Hall, a world-renowned destination spa, on a midweek break for two. Mum finished writing a book not that long ago and I promised her a spa as a treat. It's supposed to be a treat for me too, and I have come to see it as part of my preparation for the Indoor Tennis Centre Spring Open. I will play tennis each morning and be massaged each afternoon. I will do circuits in the gym and warm my muscles in the sauna. I intend to feel a bit like Nadal, but without the neuroses.

Eventually the LTA page refreshes properly, and the ratings run is complete. In my age group (40+) I am number 21 in Kent and 311 in Britain. Without taking my age into account, I am 75th in Kent and 1,690th in Britain. I am both delighted and bewildered. Of course it means nothing, I tell myself. So few women over forty even play singles, let alone travel to tournaments to play singles. But I decide that by the end of this year I want to be number 1 in Kent in my age group. In the end, this might be about who plays the most tournaments. Well, so be it. Game on.

•

Normal British people do not look better in dressing gowns with no makeup and their hair scraped back. They may feel more relaxed like that, but I do not feel relaxed watching them. The fact that I hate myself a bit for feeling like this is also not relaxing. They laugh. They cough. They distract me from my mindfulness book. I particularly hate watching them eat. I imagine spending all day in a dressing gown that smells of lunch and has gravy stains from dinner. It costs £3.50 to rent a dressing gown at Ragdale Hall, a sum surely easier to add to the cost of a room for the night (approximately £175) than charge on an item-by-item basis, involving attaching off-putting paper seals around each dressing gown. I am on my second one after inadvertently wearing the first one to lunch. I can't stand for anything to smell of food, apart from food. And only when I am eating it. I want to feel like an athlete at a training camp but instead I feel like an aging fat woman trying to avoid smelling of gravy.

Another problem with my fantasy training camp is that I haven't been able to book any tennis. A perfunctory email ten days before our arrival told me that as the regular coach was on holiday, Ragdale Hall would not be able to offer me tennis during my stay. My response, that there surely was more than one tennis coach in Leicestershire and would they like to find one or should I, had simply been ignored. WTF? I have the money. I have the time. I have a tennis court to play on. About a week before we traveled here, I emailed a coach from a tennis academy in Loughborough. He was too busy but referred me to someone else who never replied. I need to be better with the telephone. Communication with coaches is never going to happen by email. But they've all presumably got iPhones, right? And want to make money?

This is the kind of thing I get cross about, and sometimes it's better to let go, but on my first morning at Ragdale Hall I spot a sporty, efficient, senior-looking person manning (literally) the Treatments Desk and swoop on him. Ben is sorry to hear about my problems and says he will do his best to find me someone. I tell him what I told the Treatments booking lady two weeks ago: I'd like to play tennis on each full day I am here. Fat chance, I know, especially as we are already midway through Monday morning. But I go off to the gym to do my circuits feeling oddly hopeful. With good reason: I'm only twenty minutes or so into my workout when Ben comes to tell me that a coach will be here at 11:00 a.m. And can do all week.

Matt the tennis coach is probably in his fifties. He is a stout man in a red puffer jacket and wool gloves. I'm pleased he's shown up at all: it looks like it might snow. He says most people don't cancel, whatever the weather. He's a gentle guy who plays the wrong sort of tennis for me—soft, spinning, subtle. But he has arms, and a tennis racquet, and I can use him to lower myself into that long, warm, escapist bath that tennis has become. As long as I am playing, I don't have to think about anything else. Right now I yearn to hit the ball more than I yearn to do anything.

What is happening to me? Of course, I have no idea yet that anything is; well, nothing serious. I think I'm in love, and it's a pure happy love that will never betray me. My love is for tennis and I want to play it as often as I can. I know that tennis has always done this to me: it was my very first addiction (actually, third—I had a real thing about those gumball machines that gave you gum and a toy when I was about eight, and I also could not stop myself playing *Manic Mechanic* games when I was about ten). But I have no idea how deadly this will become. No idea that I am already a mouse in a lab experiment that presses its little lever for another shot of cocaine, again and again, never even eating, never doing anything else ever again.

That first day with Matt, I love the fact that I am playing tennis, just like I always do, but hate almost everything else. I feel clenched and tight. My forehand hasn't been out since Dan did a video analysis last Thursday and showed me how late I still hit the ball. My forehand is therefore back under construction. Wonky, unstable, wrong. My backhand is the same dependable one-handed backhand I've had since I was twelve. I hate being criticized, but it turns out I also really hate being praised. Matt praises much more than Dan, but it is clear he has such low expectations of a middle-aged fat chick like me. I know I can do a lot better than he expects. My poor serve has also died since it was videoed, but Matt thinks it's pacy and powerful. "Most ladies" he knows who play in leagues would have trouble with it. And I haven't even yet done a good serve! He likes my backhand. Everyone likes my backhand. I wish someone liked my forehand.

•

Between 3:00 and 4:00 p.m. is a bad time in the thermal spa. All the new arrivals have, after their long car journeys, simply stripped and entered. No showering first. Which is sort of what I did, I suppose, now I think about it, but I'm sure I am cleaner. After my massage on Tuesday I go to the Color Flow Cave, basically a steam room with a fake crystal on the back wall with new age music playing and fluorescent light strips that change color along with the music. I like the Color Flow Cave because it is the hottest of all the steam rooms, but this time when I open the door it is cool and smells of feet. All thermal spa facilities smell of feet when they are switched off. The fact that it isn't working has not stopped some of the new arrivals. They sit there, not even aware that they are not having a good time. I look around for what's wrong. There's no steam. You can see people too clearly. As I turn to go out, one of the new arrivals asks what's up. I tell him I don't think it's working. He stays where he is.

Here is how Ragdale Hall makes money. You pay a reasonable amount for an "all-inclusive" four-night break. £735 buys you a superior double room for four nights, breakfast on a tray (which we'll come to), buffet lunch, use of all facilities, unlimited exercise classes, three-course dinner, and two cups of tea. The food is very good, especially the dinner. Each dish is labeled with one, two, or three "windows" that denote how calorific it is. Of course, you pay for your wine. You pay a supplement of £10.95 if you want the beef fillet. If you have a cup of tea that is not one of your free ones, it'll be £1.60. A gin and tonic is £6.50. At any moment that you agree to pay for anything extra, a little receipt is immediately produced and you have to sign it.

There is cake everywhere. And fat women, the ones much fatter than me, who probably fell for the exotic fruit skewer (one window) as their inclusive pudding, are paying extra to eat it. I don't eat wheat, of course, so have no cake. But I do buy a box of Valentine's Day chocolate truffles (£6.50 for six) and eat my way through those. The place is packed. I can't find out how many bedrooms there are, but I would guess there are over two hundred. One of the reviews on Tripadvisor compares the place to a cruise liner. Another suggests it's more like an old people's home. It is incredibly busy. There are residents, day guests, and locals. The locals use the place as their leisure center. It seems to employ about five hundred people.

I complain about everything. I complain about the supplements, that my wine is too warm, and that there's no one at one of the bars when I want to be served. I complain that my four-ounce glass of champagne is flat. I complain that my first massage is too light, so light it's actually irritating, like being tickled by someone who does not even fancy you. The second one is too intense. I don't like being massaged by women. I don't like waiting for anything. I am sarcastic. I do that thing where I smile and say something that sounds nice but isn't, like "I wonder whether it would be possible to have a glass of champagne that comes from a bottle that has been recently opened and is served in a glass that's actually clean." I expect I look stupid trying to be assertive in my dressing gown, but I don't care.

"I'm not sure I like Scary Scarlett," my mum says over dinner.

"For God's sake," I say grumpily. "I'm not that scary."

My mum has been calling me Scary Scarlett ever since I emerged from a bout of therapy that made me individualistic and quite a bit more combative than usual. It was the same therapist who'd introduced me to *A Course in Miracles*. I would say something about feeling guilty for not switching my engine off while waiting in a car park, and how sad I'd felt when a man had tutted at me, and the therapist would say that maybe that man needed to be angry that day and my doing something to annoy him had therefore actually *helped* him. Also—and this was her response to pretty much anything—it has already happened, so it does not matter. Everything in the universe has already happened. It's a Tralfamadorian way of seeing time. *So it goes*. Do what you like: it won't change anything. And the universe loves you anyway. However much of a massive cunt you are, the universe loves you anyway.

"And besides," I say to Mum now, "it's not like you don't benefit from me being like this. I got you a superior room, and a better breakfast, and a new dressing gown."

"I know," Mum says. "But couldn't you be nicer about it all?"

"It doesn't work when you're nice," I say. "And I'd rather be aggressive than passive-aggressive. It's more honest."

One of the annoying things about this is that I've always had to have fights on behalf of the family, sometimes literally. Mum and Couze actively encouraged me to punch a racist girl in the park when I was about ten. I'm the one who has to phone up and shout at people. Recently some guy in a van swore at my mum over a maneuver on the country lanes near where she lives, and I was the one who had to ring the company and demand he be sacked. "I am going to stay on the line until you can tell me why you think it acceptable for one of your employees to verbally abuse a woman on her own," I said to the man who answered the phone. "Or until you promise me that you are going to sack him."

We manage to get off the subject of my scariness by talking about tennis. Mum wants to know how I played today and whether

Matt was astonished by my skill. I mumble about my shots being under reconstruction and Matt being more of a hitting partner than a coach, really.

"You were a Wimbledon baby," Mum says. "You've got tennis in your blood. Did you know that your grandma played tennis?"

"What, seriously? Not your mum?"

"Yep. She had trophies. A long line of them on the mantelpiece."

"When did she play?"

When I think of Grandma, I think of a stout Geordie woman who loved cigarettes and nail varnish, would crush wasps between two fingers, and who had possibly been a nurse in the war. After the war she traveled the world with her RAF husband and my mum had a pet monkey. Then they became alcoholics and my mum had to go into foster care for a while.

"When she was a schoolgirl, I think."

"Really? Why did I never know this?"

Mum shrugs.

"Anyway, who was playing when I was being born?" I ask. I was born at 4:00 p.m. on July 5, 1972. All I have really known about this before is that "Here Comes the Sun" by the Beatles was on the radio, and also that the actual sun came out. But Wimbledon is always happening on my birthday, so I don't know why it has never dawned on me that it therefore must have been going on while I was actually being born.

"I don't know," says Mum. "I was a bit busy."

Later I look it up. It was a good year for tennis. The ladies' singles final had Billie Jean King beating Evonne Goolagong, and the men's singles had Stan Smith beating Ilie Nastase. Billie Jean King won £2,400 and Stan Smith won £5,000. It's hard to work out what day everything happened. There was a lot of rain that year. The men's final was on July 9.

"Can you remember when I first played tennis?" I ask Mum, but she can't.

"Any desserts for you ladies?" asks the waiter.

The other thing that's annoying about being here is being referred to all the sodding time as "ladies."

•

The next day Matt has plenty to say about ladies himself. It's extremely windy and he wants to teach me drop shots.

"A good shot for ladies' matches," he says.

"Can't we just hit?" I say. But he's planned a whole session around drop shots and playing in the wind and I don't want to hurt his feelings. I have come to this session imagining that I will ask Matt to make me hit my forehands higher like Azarenka, or even Becky Carter. But whatever. We can do drop shots.

Doing something I am not invested in has its advantages. I forget to be nervous. I hit the ball better. It feels free and playful. At one end the wind is such that you smack the ball and it virtually becomes a drop shot anyway. From the other end a drop shot is more than likely to go long. There are different strategies at each end. The wind somehow means I can relax and learn and have a laugh. Matt teaches me a backhand drop shot, for use into the wind against someone I've pushed back with the previous shot. I have never learned a backhand drop shot. It comes easily because I already have such a good backhand slice. "I like your backhand," Matt says again. "It's really very good." And my backhand drop shot does come more easily than the forehand. *How does this make me special?* asks a voice inside me. I need to be special. But what if my need to be special is ruining my game? In the sauna later, I will tell Mum that I love tennis more than writing, more than wine, more than almost anything. But do I love it more than being special?

Then, as it begins to sleet lightly, we do volleys. I love volleying. I actually win our little game of serve-volley, 11–9. Then Matt comes in to the net and we volley back and forth, quick and fast. He seems surprised by how confident I am. Only the "top ladies" at his club, he assures me, would feel at all comfortable doing what I am doing. I'm not sure whether to find this complimentary or just patronizing.

•

Later that evening I fetch the remains of yesterday's bottle of Châteauneuf-du-Pape from the kitchen. It's a long walk from here back to where my mother likes to sit, near the door to the smokers' area, and I do get some funny looks. No one else is walking around the spa with a half-empty bottle of red wine. But then no one uses the tennis courts either. And no one approaches the gym the way I do either, doing proper circuits and using the actual weights. I feel alive. Here we are, me with my wine and Mum with her fags, talking about how to incorporate mindfulness into tennis and life. Mum has suggested that I consider using mindfulness to help me—she was watching me play with Matt from the window, it turns out, and she was surprised to see that I wasn't completely thrashing him. Also, she wonders, what kind of second serve am I doing? Is it a kicker? She thinks it might not be "heavy" enough.

"I don't even know what that means," I say. "Where do you get this stuff from?"

"I've been watching tennis since before you were born," she says. "Just not during."

"No. Anyway, I do think mindfulness is the answer."

"I'm not arguing," I say, grumpily. Mindfulness used to be my sort of thing. I'm the hippie in the family. But recently Mum has done a course on it and now she's the expert. "It's not like I don't try."

"I could lend you a book on it."

"I already have a thousand bloody books on mindfulness," I say. "But thank you anyway. And *The Inner Game of Tennis*. Do you know about that?"

"No. What is it?"

The Inner Game of Tennis explains that you have two selves: Self 1 and Self 2. I tell Mum that Self 1 is your controlling, petty, clenched little conscious self that is driven by ego and does everything wrong because it thinks too much. Self 2 is the unconscious wise thing that quietly controls everything in the background. It's like the difference between the ego and the higher self—or, in another sports psychology book, the chimp and the human (or, perhaps more accurately, the computer). I have come across this idea a lot in my reading over the years. It's part of the Hindu philosophy I've encountered while doing yoga, the Buddhism I've drifted in and out of over the years, and even some of the forms of Christianity I've encountered, although usually that's more about a trinity than a duality.

But it's the same message anyway: Relax. Stop trying. Embrace paradox.

"And then you can become number one in the country!" Mum says. "And, who knows, maybe even the world."

•

I had a fun dinner with the writer Naomi Alderman last weekend and I've saved up some snippets from that to entertain my mother. For example, I tell her, there are people out there who write fan fiction, which is like—OK, she knows what fan fiction is—but anyway there is a kind of fan fiction called Johnlock, in which Sherlock from the BBC series and his sidekick John Watson have sex. It is all written by women. Why? asks Mum. I shrug. To express their sexuality. To be feminist in the new way. We get to talking about feminism in the new way—all that stuff about checking your privilege, and the recent debates over who on the spectrum of female is the most authentically female, and Mum tells me about how *Spare Rib* magazine was always on the verge of closing down because the women who wrote for it were too busy competing over who was the most oppressed.

Back in my room I think about the conversation I had with Naomi over breakfast the morning after the dinner. She is now working at Bath Spa University, recently taken on as professor. Professor! And she doesn't seem that far into her thirties. I have been working my way up to a chair for the last ten years, rather in the way I plan to work my way through tennis rankings now.

Naomi has made a million-selling app and been involved in advertising. I've just written books (she has also written books). Over gluten-free bagels that morning I began to tell her what I hate about my job. When I started explaining that I rarely read first novels now because they remind me of student work, which I have grown to hate, and how I clock-watch during seminars and really don't care if any of my students (save a small handful) get published or, really, whether they live or die (this isn't strictly true but I'm trying to set the mood), Naomi declared me burnt out. Maybe she was right.

She offered to put me in touch with a guy high up in an adver-

tising firm who apparently bought copies of my novel *PopCo* for all
his employees and told them that this was the kind of company he
wanted them to be. Last year I went through a phase of wanting to
leave the university and work in TV, but I couldn't find the way in.
Could I work in advertising? Not sure. Probably not. *PopCo* was my
anti-capitalist book. Who would do that? Then Naomi made the
e-introductions and then the advertising guy got in touch to tell me
he loved my books. I have, so far, done nothing. It's late here, but
he's in America, where it is not late. I'm a bit drunk. I email him
saying I want to do something more "stimulating and evil" than
work in a university. I tell him I'm bored with my job and looking
for something else. I tell him I love his showreel. Not thinking, I use
my University of Kent email account to send the message.

•

Thursday morning is bright and clear and cold. I have developed
a sore throat overnight. I rarely get colds, especially at this time of
year. Is it because of playing outside so much in the wind and sleet?
But Matt seems fine and he does it all the time. Reluctantly, I ask
to cut the session short and do only an hour, despite having booked
an hour and a half. We warm up, and Matt says I'm hitting the ball
better than he's seen me so far. That's good—I'm trying to focus
on my breathing. I'm trying a kind of yoga-mindfulness-tennis. I
breathe in as the ball approaches me and out as I hit it. As I breathe
out, I make a little noise. It's my grunt! At last! Except that I have to
cough immediately afterward. I am pretty sick of playing tennis in
the Midlands in the winter now. We do some patterns of play and I
open up spaces in which to hit the ball, but I still do it hesitantly, politely. Matt wants to know why I still refuse to finish off a rally with

a killer ground stroke. Why, he asks, do I freeze whenever we play a point? I don't know. I wish I knew. I am timid, safe, and comfortable when I want to be hard, fast, dangerous.

I don't know how to articulate this to anyone, and maybe I never will—maybe I don't actually want to win. Maybe I just want to keep hitting the ball. I mean yes, of course, I want to win the point, and the game, and I want another trophy more than anything in the world. *Almost*. But I sense that there is a deep, deep part of me that doesn't want to crush my opponent, that wants this game to be beautiful and cooperative and long, and somehow to the death, but with no winners and no losers, just a pure sense of eternity. I bury this feeling.

On the way home I buy another fluorescent yellow bra from JD Sports at St. Pancras station. It's the kind of thing you could wear to be hard and fast and dangerous. I imagine wearing it with a little tank top and tight shorts, and my abs looking like Becky Carter's.

That evening at home I am thinking about my timidity for the thousandth time when the answer comes to me. I am playing tennis as I live life. For example, I have hung on to this teaching job for a lot longer than I should have done because it pays the mortgage and I don't want to be poor again. Although these are good reasons in a way, they are not valid. I have skills and savings. I could be doing something riskier that I enjoy more.

The day I felt best about my tennis was when I relaxed and had a laugh with Matt and the wind meant that a lot of shots didn't matter. It's the same with Dan. Why am I so intense? Why can I not just pretend that there is a wind that means mistakes don't matter? I am embarrassed to hit it hard. Embarrassed to grunt. Natalia Lozano just grunted immediately. That's how she plays her shots. Why do I feel embarrassed and weird about paying someone £25 an hour to teach me tennis when it costs £68 to have a rubbish fifty-minute massage, or £50 for the same amount of weird therapy? I want so much for people to like me and give me trophies that I am afraid to do anything.

Something in me makes me want to hit the ball back to people nicely and calmly until it is completely safe to make a winning move. I don't tend to make winning moves socially either. I don't mean that I don't win, but I don't take risks. I have generally waited for someone to say they love me before admitting I love them too. The idea of putting myself on the line, being rejected, hitting the ball out and having to begin the next point ...

Instead of going along to play a tennis match with my identity intact, I go looking for an identity. I go to be validated, confirmed, loved. I want to impress everyone so much that I can't move. Earlier today, playing Matt in the cold and the wind, with my lungs crackling underneath my Adidas jacket and my silk scarf, why didn't I hit out? I had nothing to lose—I was probably never going to see him again. In my defense, the shots took a lot of setting up and I didn't want to fuck them up. But so often I did anyway, by hitting lamely into the net, or hitting the ball so weakly he could not only get it back, but get it back for a winner.

•

Am I burnt out? I begin compiling a list of all the things I have come to hate about the University of Kent, the place I used to love so much (and will come to love again). On Fridays I teach in Rutherford Cloisters and have my lunch in the Rutherford dining room. What I really hate about this dining room is that the view of the cathedral—the whole point of this vast hall with its impressive picture windows—is always closed off with screens. In theory, these protect the small area of seating where they have occasional official dinners, or where visitors might be seated on Open Days. But in reality, every day the screens are there and there is no one sitting behind them.

What I particularly hate about this is that everyone seems simply to accept it. Everyone accepts that if there is a nice view it should be sealed off. It must surely be for VIPs or First Class ticket holders. It must certainly be Kept for Best. But these kids, the ones squashed onto all the other tables with no view of the cathedral, are now spending £9,000 a year to come here, and the only real selling point we have is that view of the cathedral, which they close off and no one cares or complains. I have started taking my baked potato behind the screens and sitting there on my own looking at the cathedral. *If someone tries to eject me*, I think, *I will refuse to go. I will make them call the Master of Rutherford to personally escort me out of here, and then I will ask him why this area is permanently closed off. And even then, maybe, I will refuse to move. Maybe then they will sack me and this blip in my life will be over.*

I keep thinking of other ridiculous ways I could get sacked. I get a lot of parking tickets on campus; indeed, another thing I hate about my employer is that it gives me parking tickets. I cannot easily park near my office, and even if I get to the car park at 8:55 a.m. it is already full. I now almost always park on the double yellow lines almost right next to my office, on the principle that if I am going to have to pay £15 to park here for the day, I may as well get the best spot. I was once so busy that I completely forgot to pay a parking ticket. Like other official bits and bobs, it went into one of my in-trays and died there alongside all sorts of far more shaming things—requests to read books, review books, endorse an entire spiritual system from India, sign blank stickers, marry someone in Wisconsin, and so on. Eventually a pro-vice-chancellor wrote to me threatening disciplinary action if I didn't pay it, so I did.

But what if I hadn't? Eventually they would have had to sack me. It would have been thrilling and hilarious. I could just not pay the two outstanding parking tickets I have now and wait to be sacked. It would be kind of a Dada act. I could go to the tabloids, except I probably couldn't be bothered. I never heard back from that advertising guy. I wonder if the University of Kent intercepted the email, and whether I might get sacked for sending it. But when I check, I find it went off fine. I read it through again. It does not read like I was drunk. Not at all. Should I have described his industry as evil? But it is. And I said so in *PopCo*, the book he liked so much. Perhaps I shouldn't have admitted to being bored by teaching creative writing. But I am, I am!

I have actually come to hate teaching creative writing. *Can creative writing be taught?* was one of the more provocative questions I was asked in my interview, ten years ago this spring. *Can it be marked?* Of course it can, I proclaimed at the time. Everyone knows that adjectives and adverbs are bad. So you teach the students not to use them and then if they do you give them a low mark. It was all very sleek and scientific and modern. But how tired I now am of hating adjectives and adverbs.

I've started wondering what the point is, really, of teaching creative writing. Of all the students I have ever taught, only one has written a book I would pay to read. OK, make that two. But only two, in ten years. My osteopath and soon-to-be close friend, Charlotte, once asked me how many of my students have had their books published. To date? None. (As I write now, this has risen to five.) I tried explaining just how competitive and difficult it is to succeed with the kind of writing I teach. It would be like Dan expecting his students to make it to Wimbledon. But then why does anyone who *isn't* going to make it to Wimbledon take lessons? Tennis, gardening, cooking. There are plenty of things people can enjoy without needing to become internationally acclaimed for them. But I am unhappy with my students unless they are at least reaching for that level.

Why? I don't know. But I'm not sure creative writing is the same as sport or gardening or cooking. I don't have to cook a Michelin-starred meal for my friends to enjoy it. It can just be some good food cooked simply. And of course I can play tennis with people of a similar ability. But no one enjoys the efforts of beginner writers. And writing is not something that can be quickly performed, like a piano sonata, or shown off easily like a new herbaceous border. This is one of the frustrating things about it. In order for the transaction to work, someone has to read what you've written, but in the current literary climate, it's hard enough to persuade people to read good books. Bad ones—really bad ones—don't stand a chance.

A mediocre student once asked me in all seriousness how she could prevent her awful SF series from being pirated—like, actually stolen from her hard drive and shared against her will. "What?" I said. "You mean someone distributing your book in a way you don't want and you don't make any money out of it? Ha ha! Welcome to publishing." The idea that anyone would ever want to read her work, of their own free will, was highly, highly fanciful, I told her. I explained that her work was so bad that no one was ever going to pirate it, and if they did she should be grateful. Pirating was actually one step up from her having to pay people to read her work, which was in fact what she was doing now by being in a creative writing MA program.

I said all that in a nice way, of course.

Does Nadal hate beginner tennis players? I hope not. It goes without saying that if I ever met Nadal and he gave me a few tips on my forehand, I would certainly not try to convince him that my forehand is actually better than his. That "it's all subjective." That a low, scooping, club-player's forehand, hit close to the body and low over the net, is more beautiful or effective than his *slap-thwack* topspin forehand, or Federer's, or Serena's. But students of creative writing are just as likely to scorn the greats as look up to them. They are all taught to Question Everything. This also now tires me out. Can't they fucking just shut up and get on with it?

Hitting a ball perfectly, beautifully, reading it and catching its arc and sending it back over the net to precisely the point we want—or, sometimes, to an even better place chosen by some more unconscious part of ourselves—this is within the reach of most tennis players. Perhaps you have to be Rafa to do it for four or five hours straight, but all fairly good players will do it at least once an hour.

Whatever this is, this merging with the universe and sending a ball perfectly back through the cosmos in ways that a robot could never, ever do and a computer could never, ever explain, it is above and beyond language. It can't be told; it can only be felt. To try to get beyond language, to shut it up for a while so that our brain waves can settle, so we can relax and focus, while using language itself, is near impossible. Only the very greatest of writers can use language in this way, to turn in on itself and go beyond itself and twist us up and away from ourselves like a diver kicking back up to the surface. But any kid can do it with a bat and a ball. And how many of these poor kids have been told to put down their ball and pick up a book? "It's so good to see him reading. I don't care what it is." Why? Why is reading good? Why is it better than hitting a ball?

My dog, Dreamer, whom I still miss so much, understood human language quite well, but she had the same feeling about balls that I do, and she read them deeply and profoundly. If you threw one, she would retrieve it, wherever it went. On a sunny afternoon in a new garden, she would happily unearth every ball that had ever been lost there, tennis balls worn down to sad gray rubber, deflated kid's footballs, the occasional rugby ball too, which never quite did it for her. If you threw a ball for her—tennis balls were her favorite—she would run after it, wait for the bounce, and launch herself, perfectly and beautifully, so that she would meet the ball at the apex of its arc. It would enter her mouth at the exact most sublime and satisfying moment, when the flight of the ball and the semicircle of the dog coincided with absolute mathematical precision, and then she would land as gracefully as if I'd just been watching a flawlessly executed dance move.

She also used to like waiting at the top of a hill, or a flight of stairs, for a human below to throw a ball up to her. The game now was to catch the ball perfectly (some of this depended on the throw, and you could see her disappointment when it wasn't up to scratch) and then either roll it down the hill in a perfect line, or drop it on the stairs in such a way that the ball would hit every single stair in exactly the same way all the way down. Her sleek black head would nod in satisfaction. *Bounce, bounce, bounce.* Then she would wait for it to be thrown up again. And they say animals don't feel pleasure. It was the same for her as it was for me.

Sometimes we forget that nature is all circles and arcs and parabolas, and the equations that make these things into beauty. Nature is one massive ball game, and we humans ruin it all with our emphasis on success and failure and progress and the inability of language to express anything important at all.

•

After work the next day I do two hours of singles with Lee. I like playing Lee. He's my age, sexy, and my type, but I don't fancy him at all (and I don't think he fancies me either). He's a traveling salesman who recently lost a lot of weight and is almost as obsessed with tennis as I am. He's got a nice smile and a good sense of humor. As with so many guys I meet, I see him as my mate, just like one of my brothers or their friends. My best cricket buddy ever was a guy from Pakistan named Mudassar. People don't seem to understand that in sport it is possible for men and women to genuinely be just friends. I don't know why that's the case, but it is. Mind you, I have male publishing friends as well. And academic ones. Maybe I just like guys. Anyway, Lee's a good laugh, and he usually comes to the Monday night sessions with Dan. And I always, always beat him.

I still have a killer sore throat, but I decide that this is it. Really. If I can't play every shot like I mean it today, I may as well shoot myself. I focus on my breath and do it. And it's amazing. Some shots don't work, of course, but I feel better about myself and the whole game. Less anxious. If I lose this point, there is the next one. If I lose this game, there is the next one. The breathing really helps. Focus on the breath. And my serve is so much better since watching some Nadal clips with Matt on the freezing cold Leicestershire court yesterday morning. *Rock back onto back foot. Breathe in. Throw the ball high. Exhale loudly*—I surprise myself with my grunt here—*and whack it.* It goes pretty fucking fast. And I'm sure it looks a whole lot better. I still haven't really experimented with taking the ball earlier, but the breakthrough on the serve is enough for me today. *Breathe out on the bounce. Let it all go. Breathe in on the toss. Breathe out and unleash. Loud and strong.*

From now no one is going to see my B game. I am ashamed of it. I will only play my A game. It feels amazing. Letting go and going for my shots is definitely the way forward. And I don't care if I lose, as long as I play my game.

I beat Lee 6–3, 6–1.

And then I decide I am going to leave my job and become a yoga teacher.

4

The Indoor Tennis Centre Open

What if Baby in *Dirty Dancing* had never gone home? What if she'd decided to stay at the holiday camp with Johnny and Penny and Billy and done her dance training and become one of them? She'd never feel awkward carrying a watermelon ever again. Now she'd actually be one of the insiders, a professional dancer, someone who knows rather than someone who has to learn. An old hand. A regular. One of the crowd. Part of the gang.

Think about it: Baby has two choices. She can turn into her conservative parents and begin the slow decline into the hideous hag who has to pay to be fucked, to be touched, for anyone to dance with her. Or she can become an honest proletarian. A dancer. Someone who works with their body, not with their mind. And then people will like her for who she is, and she will be real and earthy and true.

•

I have a routine now when I go to the leisure center. I pay for my tennis lesson at the desk, and then I go down to warm up in the gym. Everything hurts all the time, but I'm hoping that yoga is going to help this as well as my mind. I run a little on the treadmill. Lift a couple of weights. Row a bit. I'm becoming a regular at the leisure center, but that doesn't mean I speak to anyone. The blonde woman who works in the gym is named Sue, I know that. We sort of nod at each other, but that's it. There was one awkward time when I was on the treadmill last thing on a Sunday, and Sue was vacuuming around me and wiping down all the machines. I felt sort of humiliated on her behalf and so I tried to thank her for everything she was doing, for keeping the gym so clean and nice, and it came out wrong and ever since then I've been even more convinced that she hates me.

I've been coming to this gym for the last two years, and I have watched Sue the gym instructor transform from a woman of about my shape but perhaps a bit more so into a svelte, trim fitness chick. This happened around a year ago and then stopped, reversed, and now she is back to where she started. It's been fascinating. My body has barely changed at all in that time. Whatever I do—and in the last few years I've tried running, swimming, and now tennis—I remain at around 150 lbs. and around 32 percent body fat. Almost eleven stone, and a lot of it blubber. Why? I'm not a couch potato. I try really, really hard to stay in shape. Even when I gave up drinking, between September and December 2013, I didn't lose any weight. None at all.

Perhaps because I'm always so pissed off about this, I'm a gym menace. I scowl at anyone who is using a piece of equipment I want until they get off. I sigh and frown a lot. I take over both of the blue mats in front of the mirrors for my yoga practice. They have MTV on all the time, and I like to turn it down. They have speakers around the cardio area and the weights room and I go and find the volume knobs and fiddle with them until the sound of cheerful R&B no longer breaks through my headphones and disrupts the solid wall of '90s club music and melancholy indie tracks from my past: The The, the Smiths, Blur, SL2, A Guy Called Gerald, the Ragga Twins. One of my favorite things is to put on "The Death of a Disco Dancer" and just burn through something in a haze of weird intensity. Later it will become the track I run fastest to. I've always loved relentlessness, and that blur of chemicals you make inside yourself as you do something over and over and over again. At this point I still can't run properly, but I like the rowing machine, and I can churn out twenty-five minutes or so on the elliptical.

Lately, though, I've been watching the screens more often, sometimes even taking my headphones off to hear what's going on on MTV. There are two songs I particularly like. One is "With Ur Love" by Cher Lloyd. Four years later, editing this, I've just watched the video on YouTube and it's a bunch of inoffensive sweet young people in cheap clothes making a cheap silly video with some forgettable fat guy in a bad sweater as the love interest. But when I first see it on the screen in the gym in 2014, something about it makes me want to cry: with joy and frustration and deep, deep yearning. I want to be her, Cher Lloyd, with her skinny torso and her little skirt and her gold bow necklace, bouncing through the streets proclaiming her love for the guy in the bad sweater. There are lots of balloons. The whole video is the exact opposite of the middle-aged, fat, pointless feeling I have. This is fresh, young, spring-like, where I am rotting, autumnal, over.

The other one is "Call Me Maybe" by Carly Rae Jepsen. It's pure pop music, the kind of thing I would have liked when I was fifteen and at boarding school. In our fifth-form common room we played the Beatles and World Party, but on a Saturday morning we'd sometimes go to the twins' house in the village and watch the chart on MTV. The video we all liked then was "Joe le Taxi" by Vanessa Paradis. I've just watched it again now for the first time in thirty years. Did she really look cool then? Huh. How intriguing. I used to look like that, just with browner hair and no gap between my teeth. And we all wore baggy sweaters like that. I have never looked like Carly Rae Jepsen, with her dark fringe and cute pigtails and little shorts. None of this bothers me now. But then, in the gym in 2014? I would have killed to be sixteen again and in a pop video and thin. I pleaded with the universe for it, and when the universe said "no," it felt like bereavement, like unrequited love, like complete and total failure.

I took it out on tennis balls. I wanted to hit them harder not just because it would make me a better player, and because everyone would watch me and say the kinds of things about me that they said about Becky Carter. I just wanted to hit something and hit it hard; if possible, the Head Pro balls with the blue lettering on them. Dan and I would pick them out of the mixed baskets until we had a whole basket of good ones. Later he'd start saving the old match balls for me. Josh, though, by the time I defected to him, would sometimes open a whole new tin for our session. The hiss of the new tube of balls. The metallic sound of the top of the can being ripped off. The hope, always, at the start of a new session, that I was going to be good today. No, great. That I was going to be *great* today.

Today, a sultry, hot Sunday in July 2018, I watch the "Joe le Taxi" video a couple more times. The weird thing is, I sort of am that. I don't look fifteen any more, of course, but that's how I dance: I mean, *exactly*. I couldn't do it at fifteen, so maybe that was something I wanted then. Well, I got it. I've got the hair too. How very strange. If you'd asked me what Vanessa Paradis looked like in her video for "Joe le Taxi" before I watched it again, I would have had her with dark hair and a French girl fringe—Carly Rae Jepsen, basically. But in fact, she has my hair: blondish, beachish, long. That sexy, knowing look? Of course I now see there's something a bit pedophilic about the whole thing, but again, I couldn't do that when I was fifteen. But now that's just 101 stuff. I mean, now I can do that whenever I want. Maybe it's not that bad being a grown-up after all. But it's certainly taken me a while to get here, because it seems I've had to redo some of my childhood first. Not that I did it right this time, either.

•

The Indoor Tennis Centre ball machine is covered in the greenish-yellowish semi-fluorescent dust of the hundreds of tennis balls it has spat out and slowly killed. After Christmas, when the leisure center was open but none of the normal tennis sessions were running, I had this machine out three or four times. Eventually the leisure center receptionists began just leaving it in the corner for me. It's supposed to cost £15 an hour, but it's only worth it if you can keep it out for at least a couple of extra hours without anyone realizing. If you hit a ball into its mouth, it takes about half an hour to mend it. And its remote control doesn't work. You have to set it up, start it, and try to run back to the other side of the court before it's used up more than a couple of balls. It's likely that the remote's batteries have simply run out, but no one thinks to change them. I'm not even sure anyone ever rents it apart from me.

Today, a week before the Spring Open, it's Margaret who walks down to the ball machine's cupboard and unlocks it for me. She's the main gatekeeper here and she never fails to let me know it.

"So you're on until four," Margaret says. It's about ten past three now.

"Yeah, I usually just stay on for a couple of hours if no one else has the court booked," I say.

Margaret raises her eyebrows. "Oh you do, do you?"

I don't see what's wrong with this, but I've obviously made a faux pas. Margaret plugs in the machine.

"So I heard about your match against Bearsted," she says. "Made a bit of a meal of that one, didn't you?"

I sigh, shrug, half-smile. "We got there in the end."

"Should have finished them off more easily though," says Margaret.

"Yeah. Well, I think Hannah had her mind on her dinner party," I said. And me? I should say something about me, too, so it doesn't sound as if I'm blaming Hannah, but I don't. I should say I was timid and pathetic and—

"They complained about Becky again," says Margaret.

"What, that she's too good?"

"Yep. We can't even send Lucille to these matches any more. It's not fair."

"I don't think I've ever actually seen Lucille," I say. "She doesn't ever come to anything."

"No, well, she's busy with her kids. But she came in a couple of times when they arrived from South Africa. Got the ball machine out, had a couple of buddy hits with Josh. Honestly, it was something else. Seeing the way that she hit the ball . . ." Margaret shakes her head with admiration, something I have not seen her do very often. "It was hilarious really, some stranger coming in off the street—not even wearing sports stuff—and then hitting the ball like Serena Williams. We all just stopped and watched her."

"Right."

I want to cry. That was supposed to be *my* story. That was supposed to be me. I was supposed to be the woman who came into the tennis center one day, having been a child prodigy. I was supposed to be the one everyone stopped to watch. The one who's too good to play against old ladies in velour tracksuits. But I'm not. I thought that's who I was but in fact I'm just normal: a nobody with a low, scooping forehand and a one-handed backhand and no drive volley at all.

"You know she was top ten in South Africa?"

"What, Lucille? Really?"

"Yep. As a junior."

"Wow."

•

At my next session with Dan he's kind of sulky. He has this shot that infuriates me. It's a backhand drop shot, similar to the one I learned at Ragdale Hall but have not practiced since. He pushes me behind the baseline with a forehand down the line, deep to my backhand, which I return weakly, crosscourt. Dan then turns his body to play a normal two-handed backhand, which tells me to stay back, but at the last minute he takes one hand off and slices it so that the ball loops and drops just over the net. I'm really fast, but my knees still aren't great and so I don't make it to a lot of these drop shots.

"Dan!" I say after he does it again. "Stop it."

During the next point he does it again. Afterward I go up to the net to retrieve the ball, and he comes to get one from a serve he fluffed earlier.

"That is *such* an annoying shot," I say.

"Yeah, well," he says, his eyes fixed on the floor.

"What's the matter?"

"Nothing."

"Hang on—something is. What is it?"

He frowns. "I bet you can't get the ball machine to do that shot."

"What?"

"Your new friend, the ball machine."

"Wait—are you jealous of the ball machine?"

Dan's big eyes flick to mine and then down to the floor again.

"Not seriously though?" I say. "I'd rather play more with you but it's just you're busy and booked up—"

"I'm not *that* busy. I'm not *that* booked up."

By the end of this conversation, we've agreed that I'll have three sessions a week now, not two. But not, of course, until after the Spring Open. Everything is stopping next week for the Spring Open. It's all anyone is talking about in the ITC.

"So you're going to win, right?" I say to Dan.

"Nope," he says cheerfully. "Josh's going to win. But it would be nice to get through the first round."

•

The Indoor Tennis Centre is closed all week because of the Spring Open. The kids are playing during the day, and the adults in the evening. The men begin on Monday and the women on Tuesday, so what I imagine following is something like a mini grand slam where everyone has a match day and then a rest day and then another match until perhaps all the finals are played on Friday. I imagine a little audience like in the Christmas Tournament. Faint smatterings of applause.

My first match is scheduled for Tuesday at 5:00 p.m. and I need to practice before that. As the Indoor Tennis Centre isn't open for coaching or ball machine sessions, on Monday I go off to the Canterbury Indoor Tennis Centre for a session with the only coach they have available: Luke Green. I tried for their head coach, Simon, first. The woman on the phone sounded surprised when I requested him. Simon? Really? Don't I know that Simon only really coaches the serious county players and the people who enter tournaments? But I have entered a tournament! It's not enough.

Inspired by the Tim Parks book about meditation, *Teach Us to Sit Still*, which I'm teaching in my Writing and the Environment module for the first time this year, I have been up since 6:20. I have done my yoga and meditation—well, some. I have realized that I'll need to get up even earlier if I want to get in anything like a full session before waking Rod at 7:30. But I have done some. And—whisper it—*it is working*. Shh. Don't jinx it, don't spoil the flow. But the breathing is working. The yoga is working. Deciding to leave the university is working. *Something* is working. I no longer care if I win any more matches or trophies. I just want to breathe in and out calmly and hit the spinning, looping, beautiful yellow ball with power and focus and depth and passion, making my new grunting noise as I do so.

Or am I just fooling myself? I don't know. But here's what happens when I meet Luke: I hit the ball cleanly and properly and hard. I grunt from the beginning with no shame at all. In fact, I feel pretty fucking cool. I confide in Luke that my backhand is feeling a little neglected what with all the work on my initially weaker forehand. He says he has had the same problem. WTF? He's a nice young guy, cheaper and far less qualified than Dan. He is not intimidating in any way. He takes me seriously. He does not bark instructions at me. I hit my shots. Do a bit of work on the backhand. This is a good laugh.

We start playing points. He comes to the net and I send up an overhead, which he approaches with remarkable poise and ambition but then fluffs. "Oh no," he moans. "You've found my weakness." I point out that the overhead is surely everyone's weakness, and we laugh again, and it's very relaxed. I serve very well. I mean, I know I still don't throw the ball high enough, but I'm now getting 80 percent of my first serves in, and they're fast. I keep worrying that it will disappear, this new, wonderful serve. But it doesn't, it hasn't. So far. Luke is perfect to hit with. He's not the greatest player, but he has some lovely shots. I don't know how much of his A game I'm seeing; I actually suspect quite a lot. When the lights go out, we are 40–40, 3–2 to him. The lights do go out at the Canterbury Indoor Tennis Centre. When your hour is up, they plunge your court into darkness. Why? I remember hating this last time I played here, sometime in 2007. That's right, after that guy showed me those photographs I did go back just a couple more times. When an older man asked me to hit with him one day, I really thought it was because he thought I was fast and he liked my forehand. When the lights went out, he asked me to dinner. And it was after *that* that I never went back.

On the way home from Canterbury this time, I feel fantastic. It's stopped raining for the first time in what feels like weeks, the sun is out, and the countryside is slick with its shiny new wetlands. Ducks float on what used to be a small village green in Littlebourne. Near Worth, the swans now have a vast lake to swim on. Other birds seem to be arriving from everywhere. This used to be a field with cows in it. Now it looks like the Lake District, or somewhere in Kerala.

I have another session with Luke booked for the following morning, Tuesday, the morning of my match. I waver and then decide to go. After all, that's what the pros do, right? They warm up with a hit in the morning before their match, then have a light lunch and a massage. Andy Murray eats sushi. Rafa eats pasta, often with fish, but never meat (he says it makes him feel "heavy" before a match).

Djokovic doesn't eat gluten or dairy: he starts his day with oats and then has a vegan or fish salad for lunch. They spend all day hitting and eating right and going to the gym. I know copying them is not going to take me to Wimbledon, but surely it's not too much to ask for it to help me win the Spring Open?

My session with Luke doesn't have the novelty of the first session, and I am tight and nervous because of my first match later that day. My serving and net-play are both still looking good though, and I wonder with Luke about trying more serve-and-volleying. In his opinion this would be a good option for me and play to my strengths. We work on it a bit. I fluff a lot of the approach shots, but it's fun. I can feel a blister developing. I did the Bow during my yoga session this morning and I think I've twinged my back. I ring up Tor Spa in Ickham to see if their male masseur can do me a recovery massage tomorrow, but they are fully booked because the schools are on break.

Back at home I eat lunch and nervously await the time when I can begin getting ready. I am to be at the Indoor Tennis Centre at 4:45. I will do a quick warm-up and stretch in the gym beforehand, which means leaving home around 4:10. This means I should begin getting dressed at about 3:45. This means I should eat my scrambled egg and banana around 3:20. I find myself stuck for an hour before then with nothing to do. Well, nothing related to this evening. A voice in my head points out that most serious forty-one-year-old women would not have the luxury of spending the whole day preparing for a tennis match. Images of virtuous women who never wear eyeliner and rarely eat lunch flood into my mind. There's one changing a baby. Another on the phone. Another having a meeting. I quickly blast a few replies to emails that have been bothering me in the hope of wiping out these images. They flicker, but remain.

•

The lights seem somber and serious in the Indoor Tennis Centre when I arrive at 4:45. All the nets are thrown open and all the courts are set up for singles. Margaret has become neutral and cold, the way she does during tournaments. (At least I hope it's that and not that she suddenly hates me.) There are some other women standing around nervously. Margaret gathers us all together.

"We've got the courts until 10:00 p.m.," she says. "So I'm hoping we can get it all done and dusted today."

Good God. Really? Hang on, wait, that means three full matches in five hours. Part of me is excited at the thought of so much tennis, but mostly I feel disappointed. Yet again, a tennis tournament is something to be "done and dusted," to be got through as quickly as possible, as if it were a trip to the dentist, an overdue spring clean, or a spot of weeding. I have had this week marked in my calendar for ages. I have cleared my diary. I have been massaged, coached, fitness-trained. I have stretched. Meditated (sort of). But am I prepared for five hours of straight tennis? Is anyone? Apart from Amie Tonkiss, here with her mum and dad, the other players are all around my age. I made a decision not to stalk these players too heavily on the LTA website before the tournament, but I remember dates like 1985, 1973, 1971, and 1965. The other women look sporty but not excessively so. More than one of them is carrying an extra couple of stone that she probably doesn't want.

With all the effort I put into training and coddling my body you'd think I'd be one of the fitter players here. But of course I have my problems. The main one is the amount I sweat, because this leads both to blisters and cramps. Of course I already have the beginnings of a blister on the ball of my left foot. I have covered it with a Compeed, but I know from experience that over a short period of time the sweat glides the plaster off the blister and then rubs it against it. But it's OK: I usually manage to forget all but the worst blisters once I'm wrapped up in a game. Nadal apparently has his feet partially anesthetized before matches so he can't feel his blisters, which seems like a good idea.

I should conserve energy, and my skin, but I remember at least one of my books saying how important it is to warm up, and after all it's what Djokovic and all the others would do. So when a nice woman named Sharon asks me if I want to hit with her, I do. I'm shit, but I tell myself it's nerves. Afterward I feel a bit knackered, and my blister is worse.

I'm playing Siobhan Clarke from Kent, 8.2. She's chatty and friendly and, since I've dispensed with Brad Gilbert, I am too. Siobhan says she's never played in a tournament before, and so I take charge, looking after the match balls and bossing her through the practice—"We'll do some volleys now, and then warm up our serves"—and explaining the format of the match. I am sweet, warm, friendly. She spins her racquet (I thought I was in charge!) and I choose rough, as always. When it comes up smooth, I choose to serve. *Screw you, Brad!* I will serve because I want to be ahead in the game. I won't receive, however tactical it might be. But a few minutes later something feels wrong. I call her back over.

"You actually won the toss," I say to Siobhan. "Sorry about that."

How odd. I am so nervous that I just assumed I won the toss.

She offers to spin again, but I tell her she definitely won fair and square.

She chooses to serve.

Siobhan has a nice, high ball toss. In fact, both the other 8.2s here have beautiful tosses. Still, for some reason I am imagining an easy-ish victory over this nice person who has never played in a tournament before. I quickly go 0–30 up in the first game. Good. I imagine plowing my way on through the main draw after I win this. How cool it will be not to be pushed straight into the consolation draw! Who will I meet next? 30–15. On the next point I go to the net but Siobhan has a good lob. 30–30. On the next one she comes into the net and it seems she has a good overhead too.

She takes the first game. Bugger.

My service game goes to deuce, and then she wins that too. Hers goes to deuce and then she wins that. She is 3–0 up. But that's OK, right? I've come back from here before, What's happened here is that I have encountered another pusher. Like Karen Bayliss. Like Sally Foster. Siobhan is, however, a very good pusher. And I'm being a bit of a pusher as well, to be honest. We have these very long rallies during which I mainly hit down the middle or to her backhand and then when I try to do something risky, either I win the point or I lose the point at a ratio of around 40–60 in Siobhan's favor. She is a good net player too. If she gets to the net, she wins around 80 percent of the points. I am not making anything happen. I'm waiting and she's waiting and she's better at it. Most of our games are going to deuce and then she's winning them.

As I serve to save the set at 1–5, I feel about as low as I ever have on a tennis court. I am forty-one years old. I am past it. A complete fucking deluded idiot. I have put time into training for this, with my stupid massages and taking myself so seriously and clearing my sodding diary, and here I am being totally thrashed. This ridiculous project would only make sense if I were a much, much better tennis player. If I were Lucille, who I can see now playing a powerful top-spin forehand on Court 1. Or Becky Carter, with her leg flying up behind her and people complaining that she's too fucking good. I remind myself again that no one has ever complained that I am too good. Because I'm not. I'm shit, shit, shit. Still, I throw the ball high and breathe in. I serve beautifully, desperately, and Siobhan can't get it back. It's my first ace. But then on the next serve my calf cramps and I can't return Siobhan's return. On the next one it cramps so badly I almost fall to the floor. Who knew how involved a calf could be in a serve?

I lose the first set 1–6.

Rod's been watching, but I can't even catch his eye. 1–6. Fuck.

It's not just the cramp; I have been trying to ignore the fact that my blister is also getting worse. And something new: my arms are rubbing against my fluorescent yellow bra and chafing. I absolutely hadn't thought of this. And, not thinking I might be playing three matches, because what kind of idiot plays three matches in one evening, I only packed one spare kit. It's a different bra and top but the same scenario, where the top is thin and light and the bra more substantial. Apart from changing my clothes, what do I even do about chafing? Last time I had it was when I used to run, and something similar happened with a tank top I liked but had to abandon. I have never had it playing tennis. I wish I had a sensible short-sleeved top, but I don't. On the first set changeover I slip on my other top, although of course I can't change my bra until the match is over and I can go to the changing rooms.

But these are not really the reasons I am losing. I am losing because I'm playing this silly pushing game and not hitting out. *Again.* I am becoming sick of myself. I am bored with myself. I bore myself. *Je m'ennui.* I try to tell myself that I really have nothing to lose now. The match is as good as lost anyway so I have to try— *please*—to bring out my A game. I try to look at it all objectively. I am grunting, which is good, and I am hitting the ball a bit harder, but I am still not going for ground stroke winners. I'm not moving my opponent around the court. Indeed, more often than not I am simply hitting the ball back to her, scared to risk a winner, hoping she will fluff it. Why? She doesn't fluff it. She doesn't hit the ball that hard, but she does hit it accurately. She is waiting for *me* to fluff it, which I obligingly do.

In the first game of the second set I am more comfortable in my new top, but still worried about my cramping leg and my blister. Siobhan wins the first game. What is wrong with me? I've decided to hit out but I am *still* not doing it. I have decided that I don't care, that I am going to play wild and abandoned and violent, and I cannot make myself do it. Am I just going to give this to her, 6–1, 6–0, and then go home, cry, and give up tennis? *Every one's a winner*, I think. *Every one's a winner.* That drill with Dan where I try to hit every shot for a winner. My favorite drill, because it gives me permission to hit out. *Every one's a winner, baby.* The song starts going through my head. I start hitting the ball harder, going for my shots, trying to play winners. If I am going to lose, I think, I am at least going out in style. Fuck this. Fuck it all. Finally, my conscious brain, my ego, Self 1, whatever the hell it wants to be called, gives in and I win a game. Then another one. My strategy remains simply this: to try to hit every single ball for a winner, not caring if it actually goes out. As for the pain, I remember one of the descriptions of the challenges of meditation in Tim Parks's book. "Pain, pain, not *my* pain." I think Parks was fairly disparaging about this at the time, because some fat guru was saying it during a bad meditation session, but it stuck in my head. Pain, pain, not *my* pain. Yes.

I go 4–1 up. This is amazing! I even do the odd little fist pump to myself. Poor, cold, stressed Rod gives me encouraging looks. This is working. I can do it. Excellent. And then it begins again. The thoughts come back. I could take this set 6–1, which would be nice. Symmetrical. Then we'll be playing a championship tiebreak for the third set. If I went into that with the momentum of winning the second set, I could do it. Then I'll be back to working my way through the main draw. I wonder who I'll play next?

Before I know it, the score is 4–4.

Stop thinking! Play your shots.

I get the next game and am serving for the set on 5–4.

A voice in my head says YOU ARE SERVING FOR THE SET!!! *Thanks.*

My leg cramps. My brain cramps. It's 5–5.

Every time I get ahead or think I might win, my game closes around itself protectively. I tighten up. This is stupid.

At 6–6 Margaret comes over and reminds us about the tiebreak format.

Why can't I do this? My leg is cramping badly now, and my blister hurts, and I feel stupidly sad and alone and not at all like a winner. The thought of going through one tiebreak and then, immediately, another . . . it's just rather tiring. I am not thinking like a champion. Maybe I'll never be a champion. I let a couple of points slip away too easily, then concentrate and get a few back, but Siobhan really, really wants this, and I'm not sure I deserve it, and after all, what kind of idiot hits out in a tiebreak, which should be all about being careful and precise? *When will I learn?*

I lose the tiebreak 5–7.

Siobhan runs—yes, runs—to the net, holding out her hand. I limp over. She is exuberant and chatty and hopes my leg is not too bad and I congratulate her but then, really, babe, this match is over. She wants to keep chatting. I just want to die. She's happy. I'm sad. When Rod comes over to kiss me, I feel like a twelve-year-old who has just failed an exam. I apologize to him for not winning. Where did that come from? He says how much better I played in the beginning of the second set. I know, right! And then I went back to losing because it felt more comfortable.

As usual, I have been part of the longest match so far. This is because I am a timid moron who cannot finish a point. Others are well into their second matches by now. Margaret wants to know whether Siobhan and I are ready to carry on after a ten-minute break. Sure, why not? I have Sharon O'Reilly, 8.2, to play next. She's the nice woman I warmed up with earlier. Sharon is also chatty and friendly and I'm going to lose the match anyway so I remain chatty and friendly too. Sharon is a bit pissed off that the 10.2 she drew in the first round was Lucille, currently blasting her way through the 6.1, Kerrin Cross. Still, Sharon's just beaten 9.2 Kofo 6–0, 6–1, which I guess she's pretty happy about. I have a bye for my second round, because a player withdrew at the last minute. This late withdrawal has left three of us short of our third match. But I know the player and would have beaten her easily, so I don't feel too bad about going straight through to what is therefore the consolation draw final with Sharon.

Another consolation draw final. Whoop.

Rod goes home to get me a packet of mango and a fresh bottle of Evian and two short-sleeved T-shirts. I have already gone through all the fluid I would need for a whole afternoon of doubles and it pours straight out of me again as sweat, taking all the minerals in my body with it. Thanks, biology! Upstairs I buy another bottle of Lucozade and, after feeling oddly attracted to it, a packet of salt and vinegar crisps. Of course. It's the salt my body needs to keep the fluid in. As I walk away from the vending machines another part of my right leg starts to cramp, just above my knee.

I limp to the changing rooms and strip everything off. I put on fresh knickers, leggings, tennis skirt, and bra. My top feels clammy but I won't have a new one until Rod gets back. But the rest of me feels a lot better with a change of clothes. The final, horrible step is to peel off my socks and inspect the damage to my feet. As I thought, the Compeed has migrated around the ball of my foot, taking some skin with it. I peel it off. As usual, it has stuck to the worst part of the blister, so I am peeling off flesh along with glue. What do I do now? I'm too sweaty for another blister plaster, and the same things will only happen again anyway. All I can do is put on a fresh sock and hope for the best. It hurts when I put my foot down. But what can I do?

We are playing on Court 4. Lucille has beaten Kerrin and will go into the final of the main draw. The other semifinal is between Siobhan Clarke and Amie Tonkiss. They are warming up on Court 1. I wish Amie luck via her father as I walk past, and we have a brief chat about my match. I hope Amie beats Siobhan. I want grit and power and passion to win out over passivity and being sensible, not just in my own game but in everyone else's. But today I know I am going to keep on losing and so nothing much matters. I just want it to be over quickly. I want to hit a few nice shots, of course. I always love playing. I'll use the opportunity to practice something. Not my serve. For the sake of my calf, and my blisters, this can't be too taxing. When I win the toss I elect to receive, not for tactical reasons, but because I want to give my poor calf a rest for as long as I can. And my blister really hurts. I basically just want to stand still for as long as possible.

Sharon hits the ball with a lot more power than Siobhan. Her game suits me far better than Siobhan's, because it is harder, faster, more the way coaches play. More, I suppose, what I'm used to. And because she is taking more risks, she makes more errors. But none of that matters, because I am in pain. I have to go for more winners myself, because I don't want to protract the points. I also—and I hate myself a little bit for this—do a few pusher things because it is clear Sharon does not like them. If I play it short, for example, she is as likely to hit it long as she is to hit a winner. But most of the time I hit it harder. I think I am going to lose and so I hit it harder. And then I start to win. I think I'm about 5–1 up in the first set when I properly notice that I am winning. Then a new phrase comes into my head: Win, win, not *my* win. It simply seems so incongruous that I would be winning that I don't believe I am. I take the first set 6–2. All I am capable of thinking, as I chew on my changeover mango, is *WTF?*

I relax even more in the second set. I remember reading about a doubles pair who were one set up in a match when one of them got injured. They deliberately gave away the second set on the basis that it was easier to win the ten points needed for the championship tiebreak that would decide the third set than to win all the points needed for a normal second set. Their gamble paid off. *So, I think, it doesn't matter if I don't win this set. I can rest. Come back in the championship tiebreak or, to be honest, even not at all.* I am still pretty gutted about losing to Siobhan, and my calf hurts, and my blister is agony, and I think I also have PMS. Win, win, not *my* win. Loss, loss, not *my* loss. I am interested to see what Sharon does in this set. After all, I fought back in the second set of my last game. But Sharon is on her third match and I think some of the fight has gone out of her. Not by any means all of it—indeed, in the last games of the set she seems to adopt an all-or-nothing strategy that leads to some blistering shots and improbable rallies in which we both play well. But her strategy finally loses her more points that it gains. At one point I become aware that I am winning points off my second serve because she prefers the power of my first serve and over-hits her return of the second. But I couldn't live with myself if I decided to serve second serves all the time because of this. And I'm winning anyway.

Win, win, not *my* win.

I am winning anyway.

Dan has been lurking around for the whole evening, but has mainly stayed hidden in the office. I have just finished serving to go 5–1 up in this set when I notice him sitting at the far end of the hall watching the game. Sometimes I get more nervous when Dan watches. But I have lost all shame this evening. I decide to win this in style. I go 0–40 up. The penultimate point has it all: volleys, over-heads, low-percentage returns, scrambles to and from the net. But I get out of position and Sharon blasts one down the line. 15–40. OK. Could she come back from here? She could, she could. She could win the whole match from here. *Concentrate.* But then she double-faults and the game is mine. I have actually won this, 6–2, 6–1. I don't feel like a winner, don't feel like I've tried quite hard enough. Feel a bit that Sharon lost the game more than I won it. Wish I had a more beautiful, powerful, earlier forehand.

Win, win, not *my* win.

When we shake hands I say how much I enjoyed the game, and how tired she must be after all this tennis. Of course I don't mind chatting after this match because I have won. She says something about my injuries and I don't want her to feel bad so I tell the truth, which is that having them as a distraction was probably helpful in some way. I tell her I really enjoyed her style of play, with that bit more pace coming onto the ball, and she says that this is something she's been trying to work on. I am tired, full of salt and glucose, and I definitely have PMS. And so I can't help hating myself a little bit because I suspect that I just took advantage of someone else who was trying to hit out and swing through her shots. In a way I feel like I just beat myself. Twice.

Still, I've just won another consolation draw final! I wonder if there's some sort of trophy. Dan nods approvingly as I walk past the office to go up the stairs to leave the ITC. I can barely manage it, but the sweet feeling of victory pushes me to the top. Just.

The next day I obsessively check the results of the tournament. I want to see it all written down. Because I won something! I actually won something. I—

When the results come through, I realize that what actually happened was that I came fifth out of eight. Well, seven. I basically came third from last. Only two people played worse than me. So I didn't really win anything. Lucille won.

But I got a few ranking points for beating Sharon. I did.

And I can't walk properly for five days.

5

Wolverhampton

I am pretending to be a peacock, and Dan is pretending to be a dolphin.

No, it's not a dream; it's a technique Dan has learned at his Level 4 coaching training. At the moment, he and Josh are both Level 3. Having a Level 4 on the premises means being able to hold bigger, higher-rated tournaments. And having new ways to approach training, like being a peacock. Josh is the most competitive person I've ever met, though, and he's already made noises about Dan never being able to pass his Level 4. I had a buddy hit with Josh one day when Dan was on his course, and he had plenty to say about Dan's failings. But Dan is older, and officially he is the head coach at the Indoor Tennis Centre.

I preen toward the ball, feathers splayed.

Dan bobs about, clicking. The ball goes back and forth.

"Can dolphins do that?" I ask, as he rips one past me.

He just clicks.

"Shouldn't you be catching it on your nose or something?"

I preen. I splay, I open my arms as if they are my feathers.

I am, I believe, actually hitting quite a good topspin forehand this way, exaggerating my preparation, crouching down, slowly stroking the top of the ball. Later I tell Dan it felt as if I were playing in slow motion, but he says the balls were coming to me as fast as always. By then I am a cat and he is a hamster. Improbably, he still wins.

•

The idea at the moment is that I will play one tournament every two or three weeks, so I spend whole evenings browsing the LTA website for possibilities. When I first started looking, at the beginning of January, I got the impression that there were singles tennis tournaments being played all the time, all over the country. It certainly seemed as if I could play a tournament a week if I wanted to. I chose my Leicester tournament partly because it sounded accessible, as well as being timed just right to prepare me for the Spring Open. But the snob in me doesn't really want to enter things called "Way2Play" and "Born2Win" and "Tennis Solutions Matchplay." I don't really want to play fast-track ratings tournaments (whatever those even are) or Matchplay Events. I want to play in things like the Cheltenham Open and the Tunbridge Wells Open and the Salisbury Open, the last of which is played this year on March 8–9 and which I entered some time ago, as soon as it was possible to do so. I love the idea of playing a tournament over two days. I see myself in a beautiful cathedral city with the wind blowing through my hair. A good hotel. A spa. This one promises two matches on each day. Four matches! I can't wait.

The first thing I do in the mornings now is check the LTA website to see what, if anything, is happening on my competition calendar. Has a new tournament opened for entry? And who has entered my tournaments? So far no one has entered Salisbury apart from me, and I'm beginning to get worried. For a while I wondered if the surely inevitable local ladies might leave it until the last minute. But with one day to go I am still the only person on the list of entrants. Reluctantly, I begin looking for an alternative for that weekend.

There's only one other real possibility: it's a Grade 4 near Wolverhampton. Its main attraction is that it has three players signed up for it already: an 8.1, a 9.1, and a 9.2. Could I win something like that? Possibly. If I beat the 8.1 I'd be one step closer to becoming an 8.1 myself. It's how the weird LTA rating system works; each number has two levels. My dream is to go from 8.2 to 8.1, and then to the next level, which is 7.2, and then to 7.1 and so on.

I do a bit of googling. It's two hours from Euston to Wolverhampton. I could stay in a Ramada hotel only a short cab ride from the venue. With only hours to go before the Salisbury Open closes for entries, I gulp and press the "Withdraw" button, hating this idea that I have to withdraw from a tournament I really want to play, and not quite believing that I am literally the only person in the world who wants to play it. Within minutes my £15 tournament entry fee has been refunded into my PayPal account. Then I enter Wolverhampton. I know Rod won't come with me—he understandably seems to have little desire to visit either the East or the West Midlands—and so I'll be spending another weekend in a hotel room on my own. Oh, well. It's all for the book. And I still get the most amazing thrill when the email comes through saying that my entry has been received.

I start looking ahead, getting all possible future tournaments onto my LTA website watchlist and poking around to see who is entering what. It is clear that the Grade 1 tournaments are by far the most popular. An upcoming Aegon British Tour event at Warwick has twenty players in its main draw, all with ratings of between 1.1

and 3.2. There's a further sixteen in a qualifying round, nine reserves, and ten who have withdrawn. The lowest-rated player on the reserve list is 5.2. An upcoming Grade 2 in Bolton has forty-seven entries. A 10.2 has entered that, although most of the entrants are 3s and 4s. At this moment I am too scared to enter a Grade 2, although I expect this will soon change. But I am also no longer interested in Grade 5 or 6 tournaments. This is not just because they are lame, local affairs but also because they are the ones that don't seem to attract anyone.

I can't play anything on the weekend of March 15–16 because Mum and Couze are launching a book and then I am taking my Writing and the Environment MA students on their annual country ramble. But the week after there is a tournament in Bath that I like the look of. It's a Grade 4 with no entrants yet. It's open for entries and so, click-happy, I enter. My mind immediately begins to prepare for my upcoming tournaments. I'll need hotels and train tickets. Three clean tennis outfits packed in my bag. A nutrition plan. Game plans. It's so fucking exciting I could die.

My body, meanwhile, is on the verge of not being able to take all this. Each time one thing is fixed, another thing breaks. There are those relaxation exercises you can do where you contemplate your body from your feet up to the top of your head. Indeed, this is often the way a yoga practice will end. Once at the 7:00 a.m. yoga class on holiday somewhere, the young teacher sang timidly, "My feet are relaxed. Relaxed are my feet," and continued up the body sounding at any moment as if she might burst into tears. She pronounced the word "buttocks" weirdly and then I wanted to laugh. Then I hated myself for wanting to laugh and decided I just wanted to cry too.

Anyway, my feet are not relaxed. I took advantage of the winter sales at the beginning of January and ordered a new pair of Adidas tennis shoes. I'd only been wearing them for around forty minutes when Dan ripped a crosscourt forehand so fast and so angled that in trying to retrieve it I almost collided with the net separating Courts 1 and 2. In order to not do this I had to go from running very fast to stopping very quickly. My left foot slammed into the front of my new tennis shoe and the pain was so intense that I crumpled to the floor, swearing quietly. Dan asked, not for the first time, "Have I broken you?" No, not entirely, not yet. But was my big toe broken? I wasn't sure. All I knew was that it hurt like hell.

The nail immediately went black, completely and deeply black, with perhaps just a tinge of thundercloud purple. I wrapped it in Carnation Animal Wool and managed to play tennis on it the next day, but a couple of days later I couldn't even get a shoe on. I could not walk or drive. Reluctantly I went to the doctor, but provincial NHS doctors are simply not interested in injuries sustained by the middle classes having fun. "You did this playing tennis?" was just about all she said, witheringly, before sending me to Minor Injuries at the local hospital. Apparently they would have a special needle for draining the toenail.

"A needle?" laughed the jolly fat nurse when I was eventually seen. "No, no, what you need is one of these." She got out something that looked like a huge Band-Aid and cut it in half. She drew a diagram with her ballpoint pen on the other half to show me how to cut it when I had to change the dressing, which would be three days later. But this was no normal dressing. She explained that it would draw all the "gross stuff" out of my toe. It would also relieve the pain. Great. Fantastic. Could I have another one?

"You'll be all right. You only need one change."

"But what if I do it wrong or something? Can I have another one just in case?"

"You'll be fine with that one."

I couldn't quite believe that they would not give me another dressing. I thought about how much I pay in tax every year, how many times I have wept over my tax bill. Surely they can stretch to a bloody dressing? But that is not how things work. When I got home I googled what it said on the packaging: DUODERM EXTRA THIN HYDROCOLLOID DRESSING. Of course they sell them on Amazon. Is there anything they don't sell on Amazon? "For use on post-surgical wounds, lightly exuding traumatic wounds and superficial pressure sores." I ordered two packets, just in case.

It is now March and my toenail is still black and still hurts when I sit in the Vajrasana yoga pose, which is basically kneeling, splaying your legs, and then lying backward. But it's fine to play tennis. And it turns out that my Asics Speed Gels are just the thing. They are soft, fast, kind to my toenails. And now I have attached these lovely blue shiny patches to the inners and it turns out that these little things—Engo Blister Prevention Patches—actually do prevent blisters. My feet are now fine. But my Achilles tendons are not happy. I have micro tears in my right calf. My left calf is tight. My knees are fine as long as I am running, jumping, stretching, or sitting completely still. At all other times—basically during all everyday life activities like walking up the stairs—I feel like a very old person. I squat without thinking—to get milk from the fridge, or to look at the bottom row of books in a shop—and sometimes I actually can't get up again. My quads are lovely: big, strong, and reliable. They are also prone to contracting a lot when I have finished using them, which is what puts the pressure on my knees. My friend and Pilates teacher Emma Lee always laughs and calls them thunder thighs. "You could take over the world with those!" she often assures me.

Until recently my sacroiliac joint has been giving me no end of problems, but lately it has started responding to my osteopath Charlotte Webb's attentions and also all the yoga I've been doing. Rocking Child is particularly soothing. And Vajrasana, when I can bear the pressure on my toenail. The rest of my back seems OK, and although I have a nerve that is prone to getting trapped in my right shoulder, the tennis seems actually to be helping that. My left arm is fine. It would be: I have a one-handed backhand, so it never has to do anything apart from occasionally pointing at the ball. Or tossing the ball for my serve. Actually, it doesn't like weightlifting, but seems to be over its last wrist strain. My right wrist is a bit sore from volleying practice, but squeezing a squash ball seems to help. That's it. It doesn't actually look that bad written down. My top half is basically OK. Or maybe I have just forgotten what normal is.

When I turn up for training on Tuesday, Dan has strung my new racquet. Fuck, it feels good hitting the ball with it. The strings have more bite. They chew over the ball, sending it spinning across the net in all sorts of new and complicated ways. But the best thing is that a higher tension means I can hit the ball a lot harder and it will stay in. This must be why the pros tend to go for higher tensions. They don't need more power from a racquet; they need more control. But by the end of Wednesday my right arm is killing me. All that killer-forehand practice combined with a more tightly strung racquet has led to a weird pain that begins in my shoulder and goes all the way down to the tip of my forefinger, like a red line in some sort of anatomy diagram.

"It's like my whole right side is on the verge of giving up," I tell Charlotte Webb when I see her on Friday. "Why?"

She laughs. "Because you're playing tennis about twenty times a week."

"Oh."

"You're actually doing pretty well, all things considered."

•

When the Wolverhampton tournament closes for entries there are still only four players registered. But that's OK, I tell myself. They could do a round robin, perhaps even with normal sets. And it doesn't really matter how many people there are in the main draw as long as I get as many matches as possible. If there are three other people in the tournament, I could get three matches. It's not a disaster. I look at how many ranking points you get for winning a Grade 4. 125; the same as Lucille got for winning the Spring Open. If I won this I would go ahead of her in the Kent rankings. Each tournament gives a certain period of time for withdrawal after your entry has been accepted. At least with this one it's quick; almost as soon as the main draw is published, the 8.1 goes. Left as the highest rated of three, I have to go too. I sort of understand that now. There's no real point in playing a tournament for rankings at this stage; everyone wants ratings. Anyway, you can just about have a tournament with four people, but with three? I imagine it will be canceled, but I withdraw anyway. So I have no tournament to play on March 8–9. Nothing to look forward to. Nothing to prepare for. Something inside me deflates a little.

•

It's not just my body that's giving up. Dan is complaining about his Achilles tendon. Also his knees. And a back problem.

"I guess all that wouldn't have helped in the Spring Open," I say.

It turns out Dan was humiliated even worse than I was. He lost both his matches and didn't get anywhere in the consolation draw. He didn't receive any points. He lost his second match to one of the recreational players who comes on a Tuesday and Thursday morning, a guy who was at least sixty-five.

"I was just shit," he says sadly.

"We need to do yoga," I say. "Yoga will fix everything."

"Really?" he says. "I don't know. All those fit women."

"What? Around here?" I say, laughing. "Anyway, you won't need to worry about all that. I'm going to qualify as a yoga teacher, and then I'm going to start a men's yoga class, like specifically for tennis players and footballers and stuff. You in?"

"Yeah, I'm in," says Dan. "That would be good, actually. I could do yoga if it was with you."

•

I realize how tired I am on the way to Mum and Couze's book launch. It's in Senate House at the University of London. The only way I can get there is to park the car at Ashford after teaching my class and meet Rod on the train. It's been an exhausting day. The launch goes on for a long time, with a lot of talks on the subject of poverty and children. My mum has recently completed a PhD and, with the help of Couze, has turned it into a book. Her research area was the historical exclusion of children, which I've always found ironic, given that I got expelled from school myself.

After my GCSEs I didn't want to stay on at my boarding school, locked in the middle of nowhere with my bottle-green uniform and all the boring girls who were staying there for sixth form. I wanted to go to the expensive, beautiful Perse School in Cambridge, where two of my closer friends were going. By that point I had become comfortable with the world of boarding school. I felt like an insider, even if I was the one who broke all the rules, got dangerously drunk at the end-of-term disco, and escaped to London one Sunday afternoon with my friends, because I thought no one cared and so no one would notice. We all got suspended after that.

But in the end the Troellers didn't have the money for me to carry on at private school. Or maybe they thought I was a lost cause. Princess Helena College had not turned me into Ruth's dream of a polite, well-spoken girl headed for philosophy, politics, and economics at Oxford. If anything, I'd become more confident in myself—my actual self—and I was interested in breaking as many rules as possible. I begged to go to the Hills Road Sixth Form College in Cambridge so I could at least be near my friends (and wear jeans to school!), but there was nowhere for me to stay. So, back in Chelmsford with my family, I applied to the local boys' grammar school, KEGS, which took a few girls in sixth form. I lasted there just over one month. After all, I'd spent two years locked away in the countryside watching *Dirty Dancing* and studying Athena postcards of girls in ripped jeans and ballet shoes gazing out on a Paris skyline. I was primed. As soon as I arrived, I started living what I'd thought would be my best life. Things had become uncertain with my long-term boyfriend, so I got a new one—there was quite a lot of choice, after all. We listened to loud music in the common room, had sex, took drugs—well, OK, we made out a bit and smoked a couple of spliffs. It was enough for me and my new friend Georgia to be thrown out. Our worst crime? "Leading the boys astray."

The next weeks were the worst hell of my life up to that point, even after enduring a childhood with Steve, a summer with Ruth, and then boarding school. My mother refused to speak to me, instead bursting into tears whenever she saw me. She went to bed with headaches, exhaustion, depression—all caused by me. I liked sleeping until mid-morning, but Couze would wake me at the crack of dawn and tell me, "Your mother's been crying again." When Mum did speak to me again, it was to read out loud the diary she'd written when I was a pure precious baby, in which she had particularly hoped I'd never take drugs.

All this because of a couple of spliffs! If they hadn't wanted me to be that kind of teenager, why had they bought me the *Little Red Schoolbook*? I was quite a mild kid, but I'd always thought that they'd love me more if I were more ballsy and alternative. Apparently not. Eventually I was forced to sign a "contract" in which I agreed never to wear black, never to see my friends again, never to go to the Prince of Orange pub, and never to wear my favorite perfume, Givenchy III, which reminded my mother of the "bad times."

But we've all moved on from that, obviously. I can wear as much black as I want now, which is a relief because it makes me look so much thinner. But they stopped making Givenchy III back in the 1990s because of the oak moss in it. Instead I wear the most similar perfume I've been able to find—31 Rue Cambon by Chanel—but it's not quite the same.

After the launch we go to a Turkish restaurant and luckily I manage to sit near my brothers, so I don't have to talk to any social science academics. Mum and Couze are really proud, which is lovely to see. No one knows that this will be the last time Couze will come to London, and that the prostate cancer that had been moving very slowly through his system will start moving faster later this year. I have one glass of wine, then another. I'm trying to stay awake. Each sip of wine gives me a little buzz that then fades instantly.

Rod glances at me.

"What?" I say.

"Aren't you driving later?"

Of course I am. I'm driving him and my brother Sam from Ashford back to our house. I'm not proud of myself when I snap at him and tell him to mind his own business and stop watching me. It's only two glasses of wine, for God's sake. Or maybe three. But they'll have worn off by the time we get to Ashford, surely?

On the drive back I find I'm struggling. I ask for someone to make conversation to keep me awake. I think Rod's still a bit pissed off because I was so horrible to him at the restaurant. So Sam asks me to tell him who is my tennis nemesis. Good old Sam. He's known me longer than anyone in my life apart from Mum.

"My God," I say. "But there are so many."

"You must have one, though," he says. "One main nemesis."

And it's true, I should. But I don't know who to choose. Is it Lucille, the woman who stole my story? Is it Siobhan Clarke, who stole my victory at the ITC Open? Is it Hayley Palmer, still Dan's official mixed doubles partner, even though I've been playing all the matches? No. My nemesis is Becky Carter. Pure, blonde, sweet, teenage Becky Carter, with the firmest stomach, the most perfect abs, and no massive fuckups behind her.

•

League doubles matches have stopped being exciting and have instead become familiar and almost dull. I am now one of those people that turns up for a 7:00 p.m. match at 7:00 p.m., although I do still warm up in the gym first. I even sometimes remember to change ends when a tiebreak score is divisible by six. I know how to fill in the result form, and am often made de facto captain for this reason.

I have completely given up on Brad Gilbert and chat happily with the other team between sets, games, and sometimes even points. I congratulate them when they play good shots. I am a Good Sport. I don't hate myself. Except when I lose.

The women's Slazenger Inter Club League matches are played on a Wednesday night. This is the same night as trampolining practice, so the leisure center's upstairs is full of little girls in makeup with their names sewn on their bottoms in sequins. As I go in, achy and tired, to play Ashford First Team, I hear a dad say to his daughter, "The thing is, Kayleigh, you just can't win competitions. It's time we faced up to it." Poor kid. I know how she feels.

Still, it is glamorous, playing for the ITC Ladies' First Team. I've been playing as Hannah Martin's partner for a while now. Hannah and I work particularly well together. I'm outrageous; she's polite. I hit hard; she's accurate. We even have a few patterns of play that work. She's really good at keeping rallies going from the back; I'm good as the aggressive punch-volleyer waiting to pick off the weak return.

None of that is going to work against Ashford, though. There simply are no weak returns. Women's doubles in tennis is sometimes—most of the time—like watching paint dry, particularly at the higher levels of local league tennis. It's grueling and long—like childbirth, marriage, and Weight Watchers. The server will place the ball carefully, usually wide so as not to hit the volleyer in the head, and then a long crosscourt rally will begin. Then it's simply a matter of who blinks first. If you are the player at the back, you are looking for the moment when the volleyer has effectively drifted off—either to sleep, or just a millimeter out of position—to blast the ball down the tramlines. If you are the volleyer, you are looking for the crosscourt ball that's a little weaker than the others, because you can then "poach" it. Much more poaching goes on when there are men involved. Put four women together and no one's going to poach anything. It just seems too up-yourself.

Normally I'm not bothered by such niceties, but the Ashford team is really, really good. There's an extremely sexy dark-haired player named Susie. What is it about her? They are all fit, but no one is young or has abs like Becky Carter's. They look like rugby players or CrossFitters. Their Ashford team T-shirts look as if they've been in the wash thousands of times. They are all wearing battered Adidas baseball caps or visors. They look amazing. They absolutely thrash us. We don't even get one game. Susie even does some poaching. As soon as I get home, I go on Amazon and order a black Adidas cap.

Early the next week, Margaret leaves me a message saying she wants to talk to me about "team matters" for next season. I've been feeling anxious about this because I'm not sure how to tell her that I don't really want to play ladies' doubles. Am I even sure I don't? Am I just really smugly thinking I'm good enough to play singles? Is everyone laughing at me because I'm too old? And maybe doubles is good for me. McEnroe used to play doubles to keep fit for singles. And I love mixed. Dan and I have just played against Hythe, and although we lost one of our matches—mainly because of a big, strong player named Chuck—we thrashed the other pair. And I'm finally feeling good playing all this tennis. Osteopath Charlotte has explained that this is the "hair of the dog" principle, whereby I am continually preventing my body ever being able to recover—which is when it feels bad—by never stopping.

"It's basically like being an alcoholic, but with sport," she says at the end of our next session. Am I listening? Not in the way I should be.

The following Wednesday, I have a good session with Dan. I'm so enjoying the awesomeness of my tightly strung Juice racquet, and my arm feels better now too. After Dan leaves, and while Margaret is upstairs getting a cup of tea, three guys ask me to join them for a few games. This is the kind of thing I have fantasized about since I was a kid. Being asked to join in with someone's cricket game or football down the park. And especially being a girl, and being asked by guys! One of them is a Kiwi: he's pleased I can identify his accent. One's a German, one's a Scot. They always play as a threesome. I feel a bit like a pro or at least a semipro in my matching Adidas outfit, with my coach just gone. I feel almost like I am doing them a favor by playing with them. Bringing them some glitz and glamour. I play OK, but my legs are shaking afterward. I shouldn't really have just added an extra half hour of tennis when I'm playing tonight. I'm playing for the First Team again. I love saying that. I also love telling the Second Team—Cheryl, Bev, Sylvia, and Hayley Palmer—that I can't play down any more, now that I've played for the First Team more than twice.

Before I leave, I go in to see Margaret. She has a moan about Ashford First Team and their victory the week before. Did I see how they were warming up before the match? Running around the courts and doing arm exercises! Who did they think they were? I approved of their warm-up, and wish we did something similar, but think it best to say nothing.

Margaret's wondering how many teams I want to play for in the new season. Obviously I'm going to be on the Aegon team, where we play singles as well as doubles, and Margaret says she's going to put me on the First Team for that. My ego swells a little, although really, what else did I expect? Not to be put in the First Team for what I'm best at? Unthinkable. Then she talks about ladies' doubles and mixed doubles and it looks like I could end up on three or four teams but of course I've got my singles tournaments . . .

"Where do you see me fitting in best?" I ask her.

I must say that although my priority is to protect my singles tournaments, none of them ever seem to run anyway, and I feel really quite special, being called into Margaret's office like this, like I am an important member of the club—

"I've put you down for the ladies' First Team," says Margaret. I swell a little more. "You can play with Hannah. We'll have Fiona as well, of course, and then there's Sally who might want to play. You'll be a good foursome. A strong team."

"OK, well, thanks—"

"And you can captain that if you'd like to."

What? Fuck. Wow.

"OK." Swelling, swelling. "Yes, great." But— "What about Lucille and Becky?" I am suspicious of a First Team that does not include Lucille and Becky.

"Oh. Yes. Well." Margaret moves a piece of paper on her desk. "They've actually both defected to Walmer."

"What, like playing for their teams?" I am planning to join Walmer myself. But not to actually play for them. I mean, not unless they make me a better offer. Although actually, now that I have been asked to captain the ladies' First Team at the Indoor Tennis Centre, I realize that I will be loyal to them for life.

"Yes."

"Oh. Bummer."

"I know. I might have to leave Herne Bay and start playing here instead."

It's always been an unexplained element of Margaret that she plays for Herne Bay rather than here.

This is how I have started seeing the hierarchy of women at the Indoor Tennis Centre: If we ignore Hayley, who hits it hard but makes a lot of errors and, OK, *might* be better than me but always plays for Bev's team and never for the First Team, then it's obvious that it goes Lucille, Becky, me. Right? Indeed, Margaret is certainly making this clear now. They have gone, so I am the captain of the ladies' First Team, which is basically being the best woman player in the club. I relax a little. If Lucille and Becky have gone, then perhaps I don't have to beat them anymore. I have won! Something in me deflates a little, and I find I'm not sure about all this. If you take away Lucille and Becky and ignore Hayley, then OK, maybe I am the best woman singles player in the club. Possibly. Probably. Unless there are people I don't know about. If you don't count Amie Tonkiss, who belongs to Canterbury and who I beat anyway and Margaret. But doubles? I am, when it comes down to it, still rubbish at doubles. Whenever I go to the Tuesday or Thursday daytime sessions and play against specialized doubles players, they thrash me. It doesn't matter that I am stronger and fitter and better at running and retrieving and finding gaps on a singles court. They have a soft, light, cunning touch. They are unbeatable at the net.

But.

If Margaret thinks I've got potential then so be it. She must know, after all. She must have seen countless players come and go. She thinks I am the right person to be captain of the First Team. We talk for a while longer about what it means to be a captain and how some people don't take it seriously but that it is a very important role. I assure Margaret that I feel honored and that I will do my very best.

When I leave, I feel like punching the air or doing a little dance. When I get to the leisure center car park, I find that I've got a parking ticket.

•

On Monday after the evening Reccy session, Sylvia, Cheryl, Hayley, and I are called in to Margaret's office to talk about our upcoming away game at Bearsted. If we can win 3–1 or 4–0 then we will win the league and go into the final. This is not my team. This is Bev's team. The Second Team. I have been assured that I can play "down" because it's in a different league from the First Team that I've been playing for. Whatever. I am gracious. Even though I am *captain of the ladies' First Team* I can bring my genius and talent to the Seconds just this once. And when I am named as one of the First Team, I won't be able to play down at all. Anyway, I joke that I don't care whether we win or lose because it's not my team and not my final but I am actually quite caught up in the excitement.

I am also terrified because I not only have to play with Hayley, I have to drive her there. On my pathetic non-highway route. Still, for now I soak up the glamour of being part of this serious team talk. Also, while we're here, Margaret wants to make some final checks on the teams. Would I like to play mixed doubles as Dan's official partner? Yes! He's going to be playing in two mixed teams this season. He'll partner Hayley in one of the teams and me in another. Probably me in the Kent league and Hayley in the East Kent league. The East Kent league has stronger, tougher opponents. It also involves not having to drive to Bromley and Shooter's Hill, but going to more civilized places like Canterbury and Hythe. But whatever. I am thrilled to have been chosen once more.

All week I keep thinking this delicious thought: I am Captain of the ladies' First Team. I am the Indoor Tennis Centre Ladies' First Team Captain. I know, deep down, that it's not exactly what I want from my tennis; not what I'd planned for this year. But I am puffed up with pride and excitement nevertheless. I tell my mother. I tell my brothers. I go on and on about it to Rod. I will tell more people as soon as I get the chance. The following Wednesday, a writer that I like, not just professionally but personally, is coming to read at the university. There's a dinner afterward. But instead I'm going to the Wednesday evening tennis session because after that is when Margaret announces the teams. There's also a Wimbledon ballot that I'm less interested in, partly because I don't know what it is. I want to be there in person to be given my fixture list and my captain's pack. I want there to be an audience when I am announced as First Team captain. I keep my best tennis outfit back for Wednesday.

•

Wednesday evening comes. A lot of the regulars are at the club session. Bev, Cheryl, Tim, Lee, Sylvia, and Jon Wise, who captains one of the men's teams. Carolla from Walmer is also there. In the first game of the evening Cheryl and I beat Carolla and Lee 6–0. But Lee has improved a lot and when Tim and I take on him and Jon, they thrash us. All the time my ego is whirring away, making "sense" out of what is happening. Of course I am the strongest lady; I must be to be put with a man against two men. So then why can't I do better? Tim and Lee, who are my friends, I see as mere weaklings. The real contest here is between me and Jon. I lose. FFS. Then I have to play with Tim again, against Lee *again*. This time Lee plays with Sylvia, who is good, cunning, hits the ball hard and serves well, but whom I never feel threatened by. We scrape a win.

Then I'm playing with Sylvia against Bev and Jon. I realize how hard these experienced women hit the ball, particularly Bev and Cheryl. I mean, I beat Cheryl at singles easily and suspect I would do the same to Bev, but looking at them here with their solid netplay I think how much stronger than me they seem. I tell myself again that I have been chosen as ladies' First Team captain and they have not. Margaret knows my inner strength. But I am fading. It's nine o'clock and I have played a lot of tennis over the last three days. Today I have been to Pilates and had a ninety-minute coaching session before this. My calves feel like they have rocks in them. I am in a bad mood. Tim keeps talking about us being on the same team— he has decided he wants to play mixed doubles—and although I am Dan's partner I am dreading the possibility of ever having to play with Tim again. He's got so much potential but is often let down by nerves. I don't think my happy-happy-we're-going-to-win stuff helps him very much. More to the point, I never win when I play with him. Maybe it's me.

Tonight's session seems to go on forever. Eventually, though, Margaret says we are to assemble in the "bar" upstairs. I spend half my life in the leisure center and I didn't know it had a bar. Turns out it's one of the fuzzy-carpet rooms they use for yoga and Pilates that does indeed have a small, locked bar out of sight in the corner.

The Wimbledon ballot is first. I take no notice. It dawns on me that this is how you get tickets for Wimbledon, but I'm not interested in that. I don't want to go to Wimbledon. Why watch tennis when you can play? At last, Margaret moves on to the teams. She does the men's teams first. The First Team will be captained by Josh and will feature his brother Bobby, junior coach Adam, and the good-looking friend who always hangs around with them. The Second Team will feature Lee, Tim, Jon, and Jack.

Margaret then reads out the names of the Ladies' First Team.

I'm not one of them. WTF? The names are a blur. Why am I not there? Is it because I'm captain? Does that come afterward? But I'm sure she just read four names.

"And they'll be captained by Sylvia," she finishes.

My jaw is clenched. My hands are fists. What the actual fuck?

"And on to the Ladies' Second Team," says Margaret. "Which will be captained by Scarlett . . ."

I drive home in tears. Before I even think about what I'm doing, I send Margaret an email expressing surprise at tonight's announcement, and telling her that I actually don't want to play any ladies' doubles at all this year. I'm going to focus on singles and on writing my book—the thing I actually set out to do this year.

6

Bath

It's coming up for nine o'clock and it's dark and quiet in the ITC. Dan and I are about to start stenciling my freshly strung Juice racquet. I have two of these racquets now, but I broke a string in the original one just last week. I was worried it wouldn't be ready in time for my tournament in Bath this coming weekend. Dan never quite does things when he says he will. Once I found him lying on the floor of the tennis office dreamily eating a sandwich while his phone rang and he ignored it. It was a man about a racquet, he told me then. Always some person hassling him about stringing their racquet. This week that person became me.

But he's done it, at long last. He's written down the tension he's used (50/58) and he's also put a small "2" sticker on the inside of the frame so I can identify which of the two racquets this is. He's also put a dampener on the strings: a little red Wilson heart. The whole thing looks beautiful. Before last month I'd never had a racquet professionally strung before.

"You want to try it out then?" he asks. "Before we put the stencil on?"

Some men's doubles game is finishing up on Court 4. There's no one on Court 1. I don't have actual tennis shoes on, just a beaten-up old pair of Nikes.

"Really? I don't have the right shoes." Dan is always the one telling me to never, ever play tennis in the wrong shoes.

"You'll be all right," he says. "You must want to know how your new strings feel." He beams at me: a wide, innocent smile.

Of course I do. And yep, they are amazing. The ball seems to roll off the strings with more bite. More oomph. While we're hitting, some guy walks into the tennis center—probably another man about a racquet. Dan notices him and slams his customary "end of rally" big forehand over the net. The only trouble is that I reach it and hit it back for a crosscourt winner on his side. The man looks at me and smiles and gives me a small, appreciative nod.

•

I browse the tournaments on the LTA website almost every evening now, sitting on the sofa in the conservatory with my iPad on my knees. Plants go unwatered. I haven't gardened for ages. Everything exists in two rectangles: the tablet on my knees, and a tennis court. I'm definitely no longer entering anything organized by any outfit with a name like Quest4Fitness or Way2Play. I still want proper, dignified tournaments. Grade 4 or above. But of course they keep being canceled.

The Grade 3 tournament in Bath looked a bit frightening, but I had no choice after the Grade 4 was canceled. Perhaps it's not surprising no one wanted to play in it in the end, given the confirmation email:

In the case of the women, due to us having less courts on the Saturday than we originally had, we are most likely to play their competition on just the one day, Sunday the 23rd. If we do this, the matches may be short sets, depending on numbers, but each player is likely to get three matches on the day rather than two.

All this is subject to withdrawals and a final decision will be made after the WD.

The men will play a knockout and (compulsory) consolation event over both days (normal sets).

So I signed up for the Grade 3. Why not? There was every chance it would get canceled as well. I've also signed up for a tournament in Sutton that starts on April 16. It's a women's Grade 3 that is running as part of a general Grade 2. I'm not 100 percent sure what that means, but I've paid £25 and been accepted into the draw. My competition calendar is looking promising at last.

The only problem is that I've booked the Bath tournament so late that by the time it's confirmed, there's nowhere to stay. I've basically got to choose between an expensive spa hotel at £300 a night, or a single room in the awful hotel my mum and I ended up in when I took her to Bath for a break last year. I'd booked a nice place above a pub but when we got there they'd made a mistake and we ended up in the appropriately named Pratt's, which was at least close to the station.

I choose Pratt's. It's what a yoga chick would do, right? And maybe the universe will reward me with a win if it sees I am being humble and meek. It can't be as bad as it was last time.

My actual calendar is also looking more interesting than usual. The week before the Bath tournament we've got Alan Hollinghurst coming to talk at the Creative Writing Reading series on Tuesday, and then I'm doing a student's viva with Blake

Morrison on Thursday. I'm not that worried that I'm now turning things down to fit in all my tennis and training sessions. Can I have drinks with David and Amy? No, because I've got to go and pick up my restrung racquet. Can I go to Kuala Lumpur for a literary festival? Of course not.

Alan is here to talk about his Booker Prize–winning novel *The Line of Beauty*, among other things. I'd read *The Line of Beauty* the year before, mainly because my colleague and friend Amy Sackville said she loved it. I'd never really contemplated the aesthetic life before reading that book. I'd been brought up to value simple, minimal things. Hippie style. Shabby chic. After reading *The Line of Beauty* I went to Fenwick in Canterbury and bought Wedgewood teacups and saucers and started wearing more makeup and booking more hair appointments. It added to a similar feeling I'd had—but hadn't known exactly what to do with—when I'd watched my first Fred Astaire and Ginger Rogers film in 2010. Life could be glamorous, beautiful, indulgent. I didn't have to be the sulky vegan who went to the Groucho Club in a duffel coat with no makeup on, as I had around 1999. Why not eat a beautiful pudding? Why not drink a large glass of gorgeous, ruby-colored wine? It was the first time I'd thought of indulgence as a viable lifestyle choice. The only downside was that it hadn't done much for my waistline, which was a shame because I wanted to be an aesthetic object as well as leading an indulgent aesthetic life.

Two years on it's still a conundrum. My personal trainer is very frustrated with me. If I was doing what he tells me, I'd be losing weight. But I am not losing weight. I am staying exactly the same weight. I've maybe lost a couple of pounds, but nothing to write home about. My newish "primal" diet almost works. And chocolate ice cream is almost primal, right? As long as there's no wafer. In the

Goods Shed restaurant in Canterbury, where we have all our Creative Writing dinners, they give you a little shortbread biscuit with ice cream. But you can always just leave it.

All our Creative Writing dinners are glorious and outrageous in some way, but the one with Alan is particularly memorable. These feel like the last decadent days of higher education, and we order one of the nice wines, and steak, and quails' eggs. I soon bring the conversation around to tennis, and soon we're evaluating male tennis stars. Alan and I find we are big fans of Rafa; David Flusfeder and Dragan Todorović go for Djokovic. Amy says Boris Becker is more her type.

"It's Rafa's face," says Alan. "All that beautiful, twisted concentration as he raises his racquet to serve."

"Do you think he does that when he comes?" I ask.

"Oh yes," says Alan, with a little sigh. "Definitely."

On goes the debate. It gets dark outside. We order Chapel Down Bacchus, cheese boards. You might think Djokovic the more convincing winner, with his strict diet and his upright, robotic style. But anyone in their right mind would rather go to bed with Rafa, right? A definite yes from Alan, and from me. A big *ew* from Amy. Isn't it Rafa who is still obsessed with his mother, and who lets Uncle Toni tell him what to do? Djokovic is into real women of his own age and likes gambling and lives in Monte Carlo. Djokovic would probably be, objectively, better in bed, certainly if it was all about following instructions and having sex goals. But all that sweat and passion and complicated glory you'd get with Rafa? It would be no contest.

•

I'm sitting by the Keynes College duck pond with Blake Morrison, trying to work out what to do about the PhD we're about to examine. It's good, but the narrative lines are uncertain. We like the student, but want her to take something valuable from the experience: we're just not sure what this should be. After the viva I have lunch with Blake. It turns out he's a tennis player too. I tell him about my Bath tournament that's coming up this weekend. He tells me about his club in Blackheath. He started going just once a week, he tells me, but now he goes three or four times. He enters tournaments too—just the club ones for now. We agree that I'll go and play with him sometime soon—maybe with me giving a talk at Goldsmith's or something.

We gossip about the publishing world while drinking large glasses of Picpoul. I talk about Alan Hollinghurst's reading, mention our shared love of Nadal. Blake and I compare notes on our agents: David Miller is driving me mad. We keep arranging to meet but then he pulls out at the last minute. He's passionate and wonderful, but also infuriating. I want to do a book deal for my tennis book, but someone's stalling. Blake is interested to hear about my tennis book—he teaches life-writing, after all. He tells me about a student he had who did something similar with golf: he set some goal about improving his handicap or qualifying for a particular tournament and then dedicated his life to it. This seems to be something that lots of people are doing. We agree it'll be a better story if it goes wrong somehow. At about 3:00 p.m. my phone vibrates. It's a text from Dan. Can I play mixed doubles with him tonight? Of course. I even leave the last couple of millimeters of wine in my glass.

On court, I am relaxed and happy. This is where I belong now. We're playing Ash—the village where I used to live. They've struggled to get a team together. I recognize one of the women from Ash Physiotherapy, and there's a guy named Richard that Dan and I have played before, although he had a different partner then. Richard is very competitive. We beat him then, and he vowed we'd never beat him again. Tonight, his regular partner couldn't play, and so he's got his wife to fill in. She's not very good. She's easy to lob, easy to pass. Beating them feels mean, somehow, but this is a league match and we have to. There's an awful moment near the end where we call the score as 40–0 and she queries it. Her husband says, "No, love, we haven't won a point this game," and she insists on us going back through the points in the game: The ace I served against her. The passing shot Dan played behind her. The volley she missed.

"We *did* get a point," she insists. She has tears in her eyes.

"Just leave it, love," says Richard, not looking at anyone.

We thrash the other pair too. It's becoming a habit now. The only annoying thing is that I'm still standing in for Hayley. She's a member of this team, not me.

•

I've found the yoga teacher-training course I want to do. It's not that far away, and the next one runs in the autumn. I could take early study leave, perhaps, and just focus on qualifying. There are also courses you can do in India. You can just go and blast your way through a program there in a month or even less, but I'm not sure I want to be away for that long. I need to be here, playing tennis.

I need two references to be accepted for the course. I can get one from Lorraine, my old yoga teacher, but I also need one from my "current" teacher. This is a problem—I don't have one. I do Pilates now, not yoga. My current Pilates teacher is Emma, who I don't think approves of yoga. She certainly doesn't approve of big, dangerous, stretchy movements. Why exactly do I want to teach yoga anyway? I remind myself that I've been doing it longer than Pilates and it's a more obvious fit with the guys I want to work with. Pilates is too fiddly; there's too much focusing on your pelvic floor muscles and clenching your buttocks. It's too embarrassing. I want to get the guys doing the Warrior and the Cosmic Dancer.

Emma is one of the few women I've had a proper crush on. The first one was my friend Clare's sister Rachel when I was about fifteen. Then there was that girl in London—what even was her name? Zoe, that's right—a kind of druggy Becky Carter, with long, unwashed blonde hair and no makeup ever. Zoe smelled of weed and sweat and periods. I used to take the bus from Hackney to Surrey Quays on Sundays to smoke dope with one of my university friends, John, and she'd be there. I wasn't sure whether I wanted to be her or be with her. We were in a fashion show together, because John's boyfriend was a fashion designer. We wore rubber knickers and I felt fat as usual, much fatter than her. But I must have been really thin then.

After the last show we walked into McDonald's on Oxford Street, still in our rubber knickers, and I asked the whole shop, "So who's going to buy me a Big Mac then?" Some random guy did, and we laughed, and then I never saw her again. The only actual girlfriend I ever had, when I was eighteen, was an ethical vegetarian, and so was I, off and on. But I sometimes ate Big Macs back then too.

Emma is thin and tall with a beautiful Roman nose and a mad shock of black hair. She only ever wears Pilates clothes: for her this means unironed cotton tops that definitely don't go with her leggings. She's firm—in body and spirit—but kind, and has the sort of attention to detail that makes her one of the best Pilates instructors around. She's got a cool dog named Bertie and loads of tattoos.

The first time I met Emma, when I thought I'd have to give up tennis because of my back and my knees, I filled out a questionnaire on which I said my highest ambition was to play recreational tennis a couple of times a week. What a fucking sap I was then. Now I have a foam roller and a core and nothing can stop me.

I'm not going to tell Emma that I'm doing yoga as well as Pilates. She doesn't need to know. My schedule is filling up in a most pleasing way. Each week I now have two or three coaching sessions with Dan, as well as the Monday night Reccy session and the Wednesday night team training session. Before each of these I do about half an hour in the gym. I have Pilates on Tuesday mornings and now I'm going to be doing yoga with Loretta on Thursday evenings.

Loretta occasionally used to cover for Lorraine. Our old yoga class was in a primary school hall in Ash. There were usually squashed peas on the floor, and toward Christmas there'd be a full nativity scene with papier-mâché Mary and Joseph and donkeys. Lorraine's class was full of laughter, but Loretta's was always more serious. We stretched a *lot*. I am not a very stretchy person. And there was always something a bit punishing about her classes too. But I know she's a good teacher, and Lorraine likes her. And she's got one space in only one of her oversubscribed classes.

It's five miles down the road in Sandwich, in St. Clement's Church Hall. I put the postcode into Apple Maps and Siri manages to get me to a parking space by a big wall next to a dark and frightening graveyard. I chuck my phone in my yoga bag, zip up my hoodie, and set off. What's the worst that can happen in a deserted graveyard at 7:00 p.m. on a late-winter evening? I jump about six feet in the air when my phone loudly tells me, "You have reached your final destination." *Fucking thanks, Siri.*

St. Clement's Church Hall has a high ceiling, a hatch through to a kitchen, and old enameled radiators with teacups underneath the knobs to catch the drips. Everything is painted in that pale green '70s hospital color. The radiators gurgle away as we lie there clutching our thighs—calves if you can reach, which most people can but I can't—and pulling our legs toward us. I'm already worrying about the residential part of the yoga course. I've stuck to my semi-primal diet for a while now: I don't eat any kind of grain, and I don't eat gluten. Although I was a vegan for quite a long time and even wrote books about it, I eat a lot of steak now. What on earth am I going to eat there? It's all going to be lentils and brown rice, surely?

I guess I am really not a yoga chick. But could I become one? I could go vegetarian again, perhaps. I know they go as far as fish at the place I'll be doing the course. Obviously it doesn't matter: I can eat whatever they have, and then go back to my usual way of eating when I get home. That would be the normal approach, but it is not absolute enough for me. For years now I've thought that there is One True Way—the way humans were designed to eat and live—and all I have to do is find it. I don't like my eating to be random at any point. It has to follow food rules. If I am not bound by food rules I may as well be flying through the air, naked. Is it time for new food rules? If I am to be a yoga teacher then maybe I'll need to align myself more with grains, with brown rice, with oats and soya milk, all the things the primal movement thinks are not just bad for you but actively poisonous. But maybe the primal movement is wrong.

My quest for the One True Way of eating—for the ultimate set of food rules—means I swing back and forth between eating styles, sometimes several times over the course of a week. I can think myself back into grains at a moment's notice. How lovely and chewy and carby they are. How cheap. How humble. Each grain of brown rice is actually a cosmic seed that contains its own universe—but of course this is also why the grain of rice doesn't want to be eaten. Does the pig want to be eaten? Discuss. Although I have to say I have hardly ever eaten pork or bacon. Even at my most carnivorous, I just think pigs are too intelligent and beautiful to be zapped in some horrific slaughterhouse.

I drive into work on the last day of term still a bit sore from the league mixed doubles match the night before, thinking about my diet as usual. It's been the same all term, and I've even developed a little theory. On the carby, porridgy mornings I feel sleepy and slow but a touch more loving. On the primal days I am quicker, sharper, but more cruel. It's as if carbs are Dan and protein is Josh, although I don't know yet quite how cruel he will be. I never need the radio or podcasts on my drive to work. I'm my own forty-minute radio program: "So, civil war has broken out and you are wandering the fields—yes, these ones you're driving past now—with nothing more than a backpack with some writing stuff and maybe a nice bottle of wine. There are no shops. You are, possibly, smeared with mud and wearing a bandana. What would you eat?" I look beyond the windshield and see the last of the winter greens in the fields. There are rabbits around here. Deer. Fish in the sea. This is the stuff it's natural to eat. Maybe not so much the cows, but they are there too, for now.

So I should eat meat and vegetables tonight. Will this give me enough energy for my match the next day? This is the part that doesn't quite always add up. On a primal diet I can lose fat, but I lack oomph. The options play around in my mind—I love planning my next meal in my head. And tonight of course I'm going to be in Bath, and I've got a tournament beginning tomorrow.

So here I am. The winter is almost over and the sun is shining and I've got one more class to teach and then that's it, maybe for the rest of the year if I do get study leave. And that means I really can devote the rest of this year to tennis. I can train like a professional—I have the money and the time. Nothing can stop me. Suddenly, I can feel my muscles under my clothes. They are firmer than ever before. I feel sleek, like an animal. In that instant, I feel the closest thing to enlightenment I have ever experienced. This is what I'm meant to be doing! I park on campus and get out of the car. The world looks different, suddenly: brighter, more vivid. Then I realize that one of the lenses has fallen out of my favorite sunglasses. I actually don't care that I mistook this for enlightenment. I just laugh.

•

August 2013. I've only had a handful of tennis lessons by this point and I've already got a terrible back from hitting the ball. I'm in Devon to spend a week looking after my mother, who is due to have an operation on an ovarian cyst. While I'm here I'm also going to see Mum's osteopath, because the one back home, the one I saw before I discovered Charlotte, was so mean to me. I can't give up tennis now. It already feels like one of the most important things in my life. The osteopath at home pretty much told me to give up. I was forty, after all. What should I expect? I was forty, with a sedentary job and a back like a cab driver's, and I deserved everything I got. I should give up exercise, get fat, and die.

We arrive at Torbay Outpatients at 9:00 a.m. Mum is taken away to be assessed and put in the blue gown they have to wear. I sit in the waiting area and wait for her to come back.

The people opposite are laughing about something. I don't know what: the man looks on the point of death. He's missing most of his teeth and is wearing a Hells Angels T-shirt. He's a bit like my original father Steve might have been, had he lived a bit longer. His wife is large and cheerful and wearing a thin flowery top. She looks as if she's about to stand up.

"Don't leave me," he says to her. "I could be dead in half an hour."

"You'll never die," she says. "You're indestructible, you."

He laughs. Wheezes. Touches his chest.

"He's got a defibrillator in there," she says to me. "Went off forty-three times in twenty-four hours once. Stupid thing."

"Felt like I was dying each time," says the man.

"Sounded like a sodding gun being fired," says the woman. She stands and picks up her handbag from the chair next to her.

"Don't leave me," he says again.

She shakes her head. Tuts. "I've got to walk the bleeding dog, haven't I? Our dog Rex," she says to me, "is blind and epileptic. Has about two fits a day. Can't see where he's going. Walks into all the furniture. They're as bad as each other, the dog and him." She nods at her husband. "What I have to put up with." She shakes her head.

"What if they don't want to operate?" he says. He looks at me. "Last time they refused to operate because of my defibrillator."

His wife rolls her eyes. "I've told them, all you need is a magnet to go on it and that'll make it stop. When the defibrillator went wrong once he electrocuted everyone who touched him, including a French nurse—and the poor dog."

"Oh well," says the man, "if I die, enjoy the bungalow."

"We're moving, you see," she says. "On Wednesday." It's Friday now.

"So I'm off home to walk the sodding dog and then pack all the sodding boxes."

"The bungalow is our dream home," says the man. "But I'll probably die before we ever get in there."

"Always moaning," she says. "Right, I'm going. Shall I order the coffin when I get in?"

"You joke," he says, "but you'll regret it when I actually go."

"I think I'll get Pete to knock something up in particleboard," she says.

Once she's gone the man falls silent. I'm reading a book on the paleo diet by Robb Wolf. I think this might be the most important book I've ever read. It is telling me how to be healthy, and this is imperative to me right now because I am never, ever coming to a place like this to be operated on. I am never going to be those people. Never. I would actually rather die.

My mother has told me I can't leave, so I end up sitting in the waiting room for seven hours. For the first few hours I'm happy enough reading my paleo book, and it's making a big impression on me. I haven't eaten meat (apart from chicken, which was my dog Dreamer's absolute favorite) for years. Am I going to have to eat meat to do this? I believe in the science. I've already read *Wheat Belly*, and this is more of the same, all about how our addiction to sugar leads to weight gain, prediabetes, and early death.

After lunch I become aware that the waiting room is filling with teenage girls and their boyfriends. Many of the girls are crying. One of them refuses to come into the building at all, and her boyfriend comes to ask for help from one of the receptionists. Most of them are wearing tracksuit bottoms and T-shirts but also a lot of makeup. Has *Teen Vogue* just done a feature on what to wear on a hospital date with your boyfriend? I try to focus on my book.

"They say I've got to take my makeup off before they'll do it," says one girl, coming back into the waiting area and talking to her boyfriend.

Another girl gets up to leave.

"I can't do it," she says. "I'm sorry." Her boyfriend hurries after her.

I don't believe it. So I've got to sit through the abortion clinic. Fucking thanks, Mum! This is my very, very worst nightmare. I avoid anything to do with abortions—news stories, books, films. Because in 1988, this was me. In those days you stayed in overnight and they did it in the morning. No one's boyfriend came. Well, mine certainly didn't. He was revising for his law finals and pretending it wasn't happening.

I was the youngest on my ward, and no one felt sorry for me. In fact, the nurses seemed to openly judge me—which didn't at all fit with my *Little Red Schoolbook* childhood and my private-school sass and the idea that you could fuck whoever you wanted—boy or girl!—and that if you got pregnant it was bad luck but your choice and an incredibly feminist, rite-of-passage thing to have an abortion. All the best people had abortions! All the girls in the films I watched had abortions. Penny, the sassy pro dancer Baby would have turned into had she stayed on at Kellerman's Resort, had an abortion. It was no big deal, right?

Except that the judgy nurses dosed me up with weird vaginal suppositories designed to make my cervix open to make the operation easier the next day, and I ended up having a miscarriage, alone in a hospital bathroom, at 4:00 a.m. I was sixteen. The hours before that I spent vaguely praying for forgiveness, knowing I was slowly killing this thing inside me that I'd come to love in a way I didn't understand.

But I can't think about it. I won't think about it. I will do everything I can to avoid thinking about it. Even now, if there's an abortion story line in a film or TV show, I switch it off. If there's a picture of an embryo in the newspaper, I hide it. Years ago, some do-gooder who had something to do with my grandma—the one with the tennis trophies—told a gruesome story that ended with a girl being brought an embryo on a silver platter and I walked out and cried and wouldn't speak to anyone for days.

Now, in the hospital, I just burrow deeper into my book.

What is it about diet books? I find them so comforting, so very gripping. They work on me in the way thrillers do on other people, except they begin with the answer and then move on to the method. The diet book formula I like best is where some guy was an athlete in college (always guys, always American—this stuff is as specific as porn) or even the army, but has started getting old and fat. His father (occasionally mother) has died from something that could have been prevented by a better diet. The dude has set out to examine the science and, with only knowledge and his bare hands, has constructed a formula for invincibility, always something on the spectrum from "only eat brown rice" to "never eat brown rice." It's a superhero narrative— the bite of the cursed arachnid—but the best kind: the kind you can actually live. I love the feeling of giving myself to it 100 percent. The dreamy, fantasy feeling of being the case study that worked. Karen from New Hampshire who lost an incredible fifty kilos all because she gave up gluten, or sugar, or all carbs, or meat, or dairy, or anything from the family *Solanaceae*. Karen who became immortal.

Later that week in Devon, while Mum recuperates in bed, I go to a mix-in session at the local tennis club. I'm hungover, as usual, and I haven't eaten carbs all day. The day before, I sat in a dark restaurant in Totnes, trying to hide from wasps. I ordered chicken wings—the first time I had ordered actual meat in a restaurant for years and years. They were delicious, but I couldn't eat them. I felt like a ravenous beast: uncivilized, unpoetic. I was eating the remains of something that used to fly. Its actual wings. Then a wasp came— it had somehow found me at the back of the restaurant—and I ran away.

I talked to Dan last week about coming to this mix-in session. I've looked it up on the website: visitors can pay £5 to join in. "I love going to mix-ins at tennis clubs when I'm on holiday," he said. "I just turn up and don't tell them I'm a coach or anything." It sounded quite glamorous when he talked about it, something from the film that everyone wants to be the star in, where you walk around by day unassumingly, wearing something anonymous like a hoodie, and then it turns out you're a martial arts star, or one of those amazing Korean dancers from TikTok, or a tennis sensation. I once read a book of my brother Sam's—probably Christopher Pike; we loved those—where someone in a small town is a secret author. Imagine *that*, I'd thought, when I was about twenty. What a dream. But when you've achieved one dream and found it disappointing, isn't it natural to want a different one?

Obviously, I have fantasized about arriving at Totnes Tennis Club in some humble disguise, with no hint of my brilliant ground strokes and my new knowledge and then blowing them all away. I have a coach. I'm not a beginner anymore! But at this point I have yet to even take a point off Dan, and I've barely ever played doubles. I've played no league tennis at all.

It's a complete, total disaster. It's all doubles, of course. I'm the person no one wants to play with. I'm put with the stronger players to "even things up." Everyone has to take their turn at playing with me, the shit one. They tut and bark instructions to "cover the tramlines!" when I let shots go past me down the line. I have no idea how this game works: where to stand, what to look for. I get lobbed, people volley balls into my face. It's fucking terrible. I'm not a prodigy; I'm just shit.

"With great power comes great responsibility." That's what Peter Parker decided after he got bitten by the radioactive spider that would turn him into Spider-Man. Is the inverse true? What do you do when it turns out you have no superpower? With no power comes great irresponsibility? Perhaps.

•

Back in Canterbury I'm wondering if I'll have time to buy new sunglasses before getting on my train to Bath. All I have to do before that is teach my last class of spring term 2014. It's inexplicably great, perhaps because I won't have to teach again until the end of September—or, if things go according to plan, the beginning of January. I'm now going to be able to focus purely on tennis, and my tennis book, and not bother about all this silly teaching, which I hate. (I do hate it, right?)

Still, it's a really good class. Everyone's relaxed. They all have good projects. Even Steph, who said she had no interest in narrative nonfiction and didn't like any of the reading they'd been given, had finally come up with an excellent idea for a project. Granted, it was sort of my idea.

"Tell me something—anything—you like," I'd said in our emergency tutorial a couple of weeks before. "Something you feel passionate about."

"I don't know," she'd said. "I don't know if I like anything. I definitely don't feel passionate about anything."

"A film, a book?"

"I do love *Wuthering Heights*," she'd admitted eventually. "It's my favorite novel. I'm obsessed with it."

"So go to Haworth," I'd said. "Recreate something from the book. Walk the moors. Even if it goes wrong it'll be interesting."

Initially she said she couldn't get the time off work and wouldn't be able to afford it anyway. But the week before the end of term, she'd actually done it. She'd taken the train to Haworth and stayed in a B&B and then walked the moors. On her own. It's her presentation this week, and we're all blown away by what a coherent, entertaining project this is. She's gone from being the worst student in the class to being one of the best.

"When I said I was going to walk on the Yorkshire moors on my own, my parents were worried I would die," says Steph, with a new sparkle in her eyes.

"When I said I was going to Dungeness, my mother seriously thought I was going there to kill myself," says Matt. He's presenting this week as well. He's another weak student who's pulled something amazing out of the bag.

I look around the room and I'm so proud of them. And we've actually had a laugh this term. I used to overprepare, fuss over what I was going to teach, worry about the students too much. This term I have taken the most laid-back approach possible. After all, I've been more interested in my tennis book and my tournaments and my coaching sessions. And I'm giving all this up, right? So when the students ask me when the deadline is for their final assignments, my response is, "How am I supposed to know? Look on the website." When one of them says they have trouble completing projects, I shrug and say, "Great. One less thing for me to mark." Each week I've gone in with my cup of tea, sat back in my chair, and told them: "Entertain me. Talk about the reading in an interesting way. I'm contributing nothing." And they have. It's probably the best class I've ever had. My lack of engagement has allowed them to relax somehow. The lack of expectation has made it possible for people to shine. Huh.

I'm feeling dreamy and blissful anyway, for some reason I can't fathom. Is it all the meditation and yoga? Everything seems happy and funny and light. And today I don't even get a parking ticket, despite being on the double yellow lines as usual. I drive straight from my class to the Canterbury train station, where I park in one of the commuter spots that no one will need until Monday and then get on the train for London. At Paddington I get a small bottle of white wine from M&S and it's the most delicious thing ever, sitting in my First Class seat on the train drinking wine with a tennis tournament ahead of me, and almost a whole year of tennis still in front of me.

Obviously, I know I'm going to lose. I've talked to Dan about it. In our session on Wednesday, I asked him how I was going to beat eighteen-year-old girls who've played about 300 tournaments each. He'd shrugged. "You're not," he said. "But you might learn something." That session was one of the best I've had with Dan. I even served an ace, my first one against him. And when we played a set I even took it to 4–3 before he won 6–4. I was one point away from going 5–3 up! Gradually, slowly, I am getting somewhere. And anyway, results don't matter. I love the feel of my tennis racquet in my hands, the rasp of my new strings, the chalky smell of the grip, and especially the way my breathing sounds when I'm on my own in the ITC, surrounded by the green of the acrylic courts.

•

Pratt's Hotel really is a joke. It's only a couple of minutes' walk from the train station and right by Yak Yeti Yak, the Tibetan restaurant where I'm planning to have dinner. I try to be amused by the chintzy, floral, ancient dayroom that looks like a residential home for the elderly in which everyone has recently died. I try to tell myself that it's humble to sleep in 50 percent polyester sheets, with a sanitary-napkin pillow. I'm an athlete. I'm really doing this. I bet beds in the Olympic Village were like this. Don't those athletes have to share rooms? Humble is good. Brutal is good. It's all fine. And it's super cheap, less than £300 for two nights. The other hotel I was looking at had a spa, but I haven't got time for a spa anyway, and it was £350 a night.

I've booked two nights because I still have no idea when I'm playing. My first match is at 10:00 a.m. on Saturday, and the final is on Sunday. It is extremely unlikely I'll make it to the final, but you never know. I've hit some awesome shots against Dan lately. And I was a child prodigy. Maybe everyone else will die except for me and the one person I could possibly beat.

I've been looking at the Yak Yeti Yak menu on the train. I've been there only once before, despite coming to Bath quite a lot. It's my mum's favorite weekend-break destination, and Rod and I came here for a sad, alcohol-infused ten days not long after Dreamer died. On that trip, I couldn't stop drinking and crying. The only thing that made life worth living was my first glass of wine of the day. I'm so glad I don't live like that anymore. Yak Yeti Yak is the kind of place my ex-vegan self would have loved. It has lentil dishes galore, but that stuff is poison, right? It certainly always makes me bloated. So what's left? Meat and vegetables. I still have some lingering vegetarian food rules, though. Lambs and ducks are too cute to eat. Pigs are too intelligent. That leaves beef or chicken, and I am always drawn to beef and then feel guilty for eating it, even after all these years.

What would a real athlete eat? I've no idea.

I order a single gin and tonic and a beef stir-fry. My drink has barely any alcohol at all, but is nicely sweet. Fizzy. My stir-fry is nice, but has a lot of onions and not enough chili. I ask for more, not sure whether I sound like a total dick. I enjoy my cauliflower with peas. I'm reading *Serious* by John McEnroe, the book held open by the salt cellar on one side and my phone on the other.

Back in my tiny hotel room I am busy, so busy. I have to meditate and stretch and set out my clothes for the next day. I have to speed-read parts of books I have bought recently, called things like *You're Trying Too Hard.* What I really need to do is try much harder to try less hard. Then, maybe, I could win? My first match is at 10:00 a.m., but I'm not quite sure how far away the university campus is. The tournament is being held in their "Sports Training Village," which sounds glamorous and terrifying. They've said "outside" but no more than that.

I can still taste onions when I wake up the next morning, too early, to a dark rainy day that looks deep, rich, and moody, but is obviously not good for playing tennis outdoors. Breakfast is not until 8:00 and I have a cab booked for 8:45, so after a brief meditation the first thing I do is shower, but I can't get it right. The flow is a tiny trickle. It would be like being pissed on, although by someone with quite a weak bladder, if the water was warm. It isn't. OK, this is not the most expensive hotel in the world, but it's the same price as a Travelodge and the last time I stayed in one of those there was hot running water. I haven't got the energy to complain, and I don't need all that angst before my first match. I wash as best I can, tell myself McEnroe would have had it worse in the 1980s, and get dressed.

I am there much too early, as always. The only address I have is for the Sports Training Village, so I get the taxi to drop me there. At the reception they have never heard of the tournament I have entered. I tell them it's a Grade 3. They don't know what that is. They realize I can't possibly be there for the inter-schools indoor tournament they are running on their warm, glitzy indoor courts, but they just don't think they have any other tournaments running. They are confused. I'm inevitably a bit of a dick. Is it nerves? Undoubtedly.

"All I know," I say, "is that I am signed up for a tournament and the postcode is here. You must have *some* idea of roughly where I might be supposed to go?"

Nope.

Eventually I find a phone number at the bottom of the confirmation email. I get through to a man with a Somerset accent who tells me that it is indeed the outdoor courts, and these are to be found half a mile back down the road. A pleasant ten-minute walk, he assures me.

It's raining. My massive black Wilson bag is heavy. I've bought it specially for this tournament. It's a bit like the one I was so impressed with at Leicester, but more up-to-date and snazzy. It can fit nine tennis racquets and has Thermoguard protection that not just keeps your drinks cold, but protects your racquets' string tension from extreme temperatures. It's also—usefully—waterproof.

I arrive at the outdoor courts disheveled and frizzy but miraculously still early. So early, in fact, that there's no one else there apart from an old bloke in a battered red Adidas cap. He's organizing his big bucket of balls.

"Hello," I say. "I'm here for the tournament? Scarlett Thomas?"

"Oh right. Lady from the phone? Bit early, aren't you? The girls won't get here for another hour. I'm Bob, by the way."

"Right. Hello! But I think my first match is at nine thirty?"

"Yeah, we're all very relaxed here, love. I'd go and get a coffee if I were you."

There is nothing around us apart from the tennis courts and Bob's shed. There's the road, some grassy banks, a field.

"You'll get a nice cup of coffee back at the training village," he says.

"Yeah, I just walked from there."

"Great facilities up there. They've got a Grade 1 in there today."

"Exciting."

"And the men's Grade 3 of course."

"Of course."

"So anyway, I'll see you back here at about half ten? You're playing Vanessa Brill, I think. Nice girl. Good player. But then they all are."

He looks me up and down. What's he seeing? He realizes that my green shoes are punky and irreverent, right? And my leg warmers are for my poor stiff calf muscles, and—

"You played a Grade 3 before?"

"No," I say. "I've only just started playing tournaments, to be honest. I'm actually writing a book about it. I—"

"You might find a Grade 3 a bit taxing in that case."

"Well, I tried for the Grade 4, but it was canceled."

"You'll enjoy playing with the girls. Nice crowd. Just try your best."

"OK."

"Right! See you in a while, then." He turns to go back into his shed.

"OK. Um, my bag's really heavy. Can I leave it in your shed?"

"Sure."

"And is there any chance of hitting up with someone?"

"You can hit up with the girls when they get here. They always have a hit-up together. Elle's playing too. And the twins." He says this as if I should know these people. As if everyone knows them. Obviously I've stalked them on the LTA website. They are all be-

tween fourteen and nineteen and have ratings of between 4.1 and
5.2. What the fuck am I doing here? I trudge back up to the training
village, telling myself that at least it's not raining any more.

•

I am now so ancient I can't tell how old individual young people are.
The ones at the Sports Training Village could be anything between
fourteen and twenty-two. The girls have amazing arses. There's the
odd fat one that probably plays in goal, but mainly these are tall,
slim, pert, slightly sulky young people. I looked like that once. I
hated myself. I hated my flawless skin. I hated my body, the way
it did what I wanted it to do. I wanted to be older, wiser. I wanted
confidence. I wanted interesting flaws. I didn't want to play sports
or win at anything. I wanted to be able to walk into a record shop
and know what to say to seem cool. I wanted to be Baby, but after
she'd become Penny.

Why did I not appreciate my skin and my hair? Why did I not
appreciate my sleek veal-calf arms and my hairless nipples and my
unlined face and my cute little B-cup boobs? Everyone says I look
really young even now, and I always laugh and say something about
expensive face cream. But compared to the people here, who are
genuinely, authentically young, I look about 150. My boobs are DD
now. Not even the fat goalkeepers here have DD boobs.

Back then I wanted so badly to be a grown-up. And now I am. Yay.

I stand out a little in the big, bright canteen. I'm obviously not
anyone's mum, so what am I doing here? Objectively, my tennis outfit could seem a touch comical: my black Adidas skirt, black leggings, leg warmers, and green shoes look quite glam at the Indoor
Tennis Centre, but here the whole thing looks like a dare or a par-

ody. I wear my hair in a single plait, because that's what Victoria Azarenka does, but my hair is not as thick as hers and the overall effect is to make me look uptight, like a pompous, aging lapdog with a stiff pomaded tail. Thank God I have dispensed with my matching set of black Adidas sweatbands (one for my head, two for my wrists) and now only wear one wristband and a black Adidas cap. My stuff is all black Adidas, but feels a bit matchy-matchy. The kids here are happy mixing Nike with Adidas and New Balance. Their limbs are bare, sleek, beautiful. They sit on the floor as if they have never had lower back issues or a tight knee. No one has their hair in a plait.

My gluten-free toast breakfast has left me a bit sugar-crashy, even though that's not supposed to happen on a primal diet. Are you supposed to eat gluten-free toast on a primal diet? Perhaps not. It's always the same when I have breakfast away: I want eggs, sausages, and bacon but I don't eat those because pigs are intelligent and pink and sweet. And do athletes eat bacon? Unlikely. Athletes eat oatmeal. I eat oatmeal from time to time now too. It gives me energy, but it's a fuzzy, hazy sort of energy. Porridge is supposed to stick to your ribs and last. With me, it goes straight to my brain and leaves me feeling empty and tearful.

Or do I feel tearful for some other reason?

I buy a cup of tea and ask if they have any gluten-free food here.

"No, sorry," says the busy young guy behind the counter, looking beyond me to one of the teenage girls in the queue I'm holding up. "Next!"

•

Vanessa Brill might be the sulkiest teenager I've ever encountered. She even makes Becky Carter seem friendly and animated. She's beautiful, of course. And she's the opposite of me in every possible way. We do have the same hair, but hers is loose and natural. Mine is not just plaited, but stuck through the hole in my new cap like I'm some perky summer camp leader from the 1980s. I am weighed down by all the things I need to play tennis: my sports drinks and my sweatbands and my schedule and my ibuprofen and my anorak in case it rains and extra shoes and extra laces and energy bars and motivational books and notes on how I should play my forehand.

She's wearing cropped Nike leggings and a little tank top. She hasn't even bothered to put on tennis shoes—she's wearing Nike Frees that are certainly in fashion, but definitely not good for your feet and ankles. But then she's small, like 100 percent willowy muscle and perfect tendons: she's never going to break. She has a massive tennis bag, but it's battered and old. I don't want mine to get rained on again, even though it's supposedly waterproof. She chucks hers on the grass. It's seen some action, unlike mine. Cute childish keyrings dangle from it. She's too young to drive, to have sex, to drink alcohol.

Her mother is about my age. "Oooh, hello," she says to me, glancing at my shoes. "We haven't seen *you* before."

"No," I say. "Er, hi."

I am saved from having to say anything else (like what?) because a car pulls up and a couple of girls get out with their mothers. These must be Elle and Natalie. They both have bags like Vanessa's. They have similar-but-different outfits. Tiny tank tops, cropped leggings, unsuitable shoes.

"Come on, you can hit up with the girls," says Mrs. Brill. "Vanessa!"

Vanessa doesn't make eye contact with me. She doesn't want to have to talk to an old person, let alone play tennis with one. But she does what her mother tells her: she drags herself to the end of the court and then starts blasting balls at me while Elle and Natalie warm up on another court. I can hear the odd giggle coming from them.

"Oh, haha!" I say, fluffing a return. "Sorry. Not quite warm enough yet."

While Vanessa continues nuking balls at me, the Kondratowitz twins, Monika and Joanna, turn up. They are tall, dark haired, striking looking, perhaps a bit older than Vanessa and the others. They start hitting up together. The mothers all have the same blow dry and highlights. They stand together and talk about the traffic, and the tennis season, and their daughters' GCSEs. They clearly bump into each other often. Their voices lower and I realize someone's asking about me. Who am I? Why am I here? Bob approaches and fills them in a bit. I hear the phrase *Grade 3* and then *Grade 4 or 5 would be better: I told her*. Vanessa has come into the net and is waiting for some overheads, but I manage to fluff them all. I can't even hit a weak ball into the air now. Really, though, Bob's right: Why am I here?

While talking to Bob, Vanessa's mother realizes that Vanessa and I are actually playing each other next, which means we shouldn't be hitting up together. She hustles her daughter back off the court. It starts to drizzle. Bob looks up at the sky and says we may as well get on with it—and we won't need a warm-up as we've already knocked up together. I haven't practiced my serve, but it doesn't really matter. Fifteen minutes later, I've lost the first set 0−6.

Vanessa's game plan is to hit the ball hard, with topspin. If I'm serving, she simply hits my serve back for a winner, either down the line or crosscourt. On the rare occasion I do manage to return one of these balls, she's there at the net to swat it away. She does this sulkily, as if this ball is a little fly that's annoying her. But there's no actual aggression in her play. It's all simply inconvenient: me, the ball. The only time she's at all animated is when she does something wrong. Even then it's a weird little giggle in the direction of her mother. She acts as if I do not exist. I almost wish I didn't. In the second set I manage to get one game, but only because she serves four double faults. She finds this particularly hilarious. At the end, her mother has to remind her to shake my hand. She still will not make eye contact with me.

Our whole match has taken thirty-nine minutes.

"Should have been love and love," I hear her mother saying to her.

Good God. I sip one of my drinks. Put my towel away. Go over to Bob's shed. I want to know about the consolation draw. Who knows? Maybe I could win my next match? I just have to hit out more, try to be more composed and aggressive and work to my game plan—

As I approach the shed, I can hear Vanessa's mother talking to Bob.

"Look," she's saying, "I'm sorry, but Vanessa's used to playing long, tough matches that last three hours. This is ridiculous. She's barely warmed up. She's ready to go back on court now."

She sees me. "No offense," she adds.

"No problem," I say. "I sincerely hope that Vanessa has a very long, tough match next."

Bob tells me that the consolation draw matches will start after lunch, so I walk back up to the training village, drizzle mixing with my tears.

OK. What exactly am I doing here? I've left Rod at home and I've come to Bath why? I know I tend to travel when I feel at all bothered about something. I did it when Dreamer was ill. I still feel guilty about that. During some of her last days she was at the vet on a drip while I traveled to Cardiff for my mum's graduation ceremony for her PhD, and then onto Gloucester for Steve's funeral. Mum and Couze, Sam, Gordian, and Rod and I stayed in the same haunted hotel where Sam and I had met Steve just a few weeks before, after not seeing him for twenty-five years. He'd looked so tragic and wrecked in his thin nylon tracksuit.

Mum complained about the ghost in her room and flirted mildly with Gordian. Apart from us, only Steve's ex-girlfriend Heather and her parents came to the funeral. It was so sad. Even the celebrant didn't show, and Sam and I had to conduct the service ourselves. At that time, as long as I had a train ticket and a hotel booking, I was fine. Before Dreamer got ill, before everything went wrong, I sometimes stayed in Canterbury on the wilder nights of the Creative Writing dinners. I even managed to get a free night at the Falstaff once because my previous room had an eerie green light and scufflings inside the walls.

Being on the road means you never have to settle anywhere: you never have to stop, never have to think. Is that what I'm doing again now? Replacing my life with an absurd tennis tour? What exactly am I not thinking about? The answers come immediately. My age, my weight, my relationship with alcohol, my pathetic slump into the mid-list, my alcoholic agent, the age of my partner, the fact that the now-or-neverness of having children has resolved into neverness, which is fine, totally fine.

If I'd had that child, back in 1988, he or she would now be older than Vanessa Brill, older even than the Kondratowitz twins. He or she would have been twenty-six this year. I could conceivably be a grandmother. At this moment, I certainly feel like one. My legs and back ache. I need some carbs.

In the canteen I get a cheese sandwich and a cup of tea and phone Rod. I can't help it: I cry down the phone to him about how terrible I was, about the rain and my poor forehand and my awful serve. He's so nice. He reminds me to hit the ball hard. Am I hitting it hard enough? Of course not. He says he misses me. I miss him too. It's only just after I hang up that I realize that Vanessa Brill and her mother are sitting at the next table and can hear everything I'm saying.

I have to get out of here. I leave the canteen and wander around the inside of the facility. It's really impressive. The tennis courts are awesome, beautiful dark gray acrylic—my favorite surface. There are lots of matches going on, some from the inter-schools thing, some from the Grade 1. I wonder where the Grade 3 men are. I watch a mixed doubles match, with kids of about thirteen or fourteen. They're a nice jumble of ethnicities. They all play with style, with proper verve. They joke around with each other. The boys try to show off with their trick shots and they don't work out and everyone laughs. I want to hang out with them, but I can't. I'm old, older than their parents. I find the loos and pee as much as I can (there are no toilets back at the outdoor courts) and go back for my consolation draw match against Monika Kondratowitz.

At least she speaks to me. I learn that she's in the early stages of a medical degree at Cambridge, where she plays tennis for their First Team. She's intelligent, mild, and a really, really good player. I realize I have no hope of beating her, but I decide to use this match to try to work on my first serve. As a result of this, I fuck up a lot of them and have to do a lot more second serves than usual. This turns out to be my secret weapon: Monika can't return my second serve! This is, of course, because it's so shit. It's shittier than anything she's ever seen. It's so slow, and lame, and short that at first she's simply standing too far back for it. Then when she comes forward, she over-hits it. I manage to get a couple of my service games to deuce and win a couple of others. In the end she beats me 6–2, 6–2. It sounds bad, when you hear a score like that. But to actually get four games off a player in a Grade 3? I'm slightly proud of myself.

Meanwhile, Vanessa Brill doesn't quite get the long, tough game she deserves. My match with Monika takes an hour and thirty-nine minutes, but Monika's sister Joanna beats Vanessa 6–3, 6–2 in only fifty-nine minutes.

So that's it. Another tennis tournament. I get a taxi back to my hotel. I think I can claim all this on expenses (it's research for a real book, after all), but I still feel glad that I went for the cheap option. But why didn't I win something? That was the deal, right? Even this stupid hotel was supposed to be part of a bargain. If I could stay in a shit hotel and win, then that would be worth it. But to stay in one and lose? That was not the deal. Would I have felt even more ridiculous standing out there in the cold with those schoolgirls knowing I'd paid £700 for a hotel and roughly £100 for my train and let's say £75 per day on food, making the whole trip around a grand? Undoubtedly.

Back at the hotel I do grown-up things. I get a gin and tonic, for a start, which sets me up for the second-worst shower I've had this year (the worst was this morning) and the third-worst I have had in my life (which involved me being electrocuted during it). I cry on the phone again to Rod. Then I do my hair and makeup and put on leggings and an anorak and set off into the heart of Saturday night in Bath. As an eighteen-year-old I might not cut it, but I think I look pretty OK for forty-one. Young guys in rapey rugby shirts won't look at me, but the older ones with nice shoes will. And women will. Not that I give a shit, of course, but it's nice to not be entirely invisible.

I'm looking for a bar, somewhere to have a cold glass of white before dinner. And here's the thing. I don't have a fifteen-year-old arse but I do have some sass. At fifteen I would never have contemplated walking downstairs, by myself, into the most intimidating, neon-lit bar I can find. I do it. I do something Vanessa Brill could not possibly do. I walk to the bar and smile at the barman. He smiles back. What wines do they do by the glass? A Sauvignon and . . . He looks. A Chablis. On special offer. He'll bring it to me. I get a table by the window overlooking the river. The barman flirts with his eyes. He is Gallic looking. Late twenties. It means nothing. I have traveled the world, loved complicated men, lectured hundreds of people, written ten books. I have worked in places like this, in London. I want to think something like *Up yours, Vanessa Brill*, but I don't. I want to, but I can't. I still wish I was living her life, her clean, unsullied, pure, winning life.

Sunday: I have a whole day to fill. My train isn't booked until Monday morning. I couldn't travel today in case I got to the Grade 3 final, which is being played this afternoon between Joanna Kondratowitz and Elle Baker, the 1 and 2 seeds. Ideally I would have afternoon tea at the Pump Room, but I also want to go to the Thermae Spa, and the times I can book my treatment clash with afternoon tea. So instead I go to the Pump Room for morning coffee. I like it when there's a pianist playing. It's elegant, perfect. But there's no pianist today.

Bath is mainly famous for Jane Austen, and the place is already full of Janeites in full eighteenth-century costume, recreating Austen novels while drinking Coke with ice and lemon. The few men dressed up as Darcy seem certain to get laid. On the next table from me, a lesbian in an anorak reads an article in one of the Sunday papers. The headline is HOW TO SPOT A PSYCHOPATH. Her partner looks a bit put out that she's being ignored. I am the only person alone. I argue with the server because they don't do gluten-free scones at this time of day and end up ordering an early lunch I don't really want.

The Thermae Spa in Bath is always a treat, though. I've been here before with Rod, and he particularly liked the sequence of the whole thing: you start off downstairs in the floatation pool, then upstairs to the steam rooms, each of which smells of something slightly different: peppermint, thyme, etc. Today I try to ignore the fact that the peppermint room is a bit too hot and the lavender one smells a bit off. I've booked the cheapest, shortest treatment, called Kraxen Stove, which involves sitting in a "traditional alpine hay chamber." In the end I feel like I'm locked in a room with burning hay. Is hay even gluten-free? I begin coughing, perhaps beginning to suffocate. Why is everything wrong all the time? Why can't I just enjoy something? I imagine how I would feel right now if I'd just won a match at a Grade 3 tournament. God, I'd give anything for that: the intense rightness of the feeling of winning. Why has this come to me so late in life, the realization that it feels so great to compete and win? Surely, surely if I want it enough I'll be able to get it? I just have to work out the right things to do, and then do them.

I finally make it to the open-air rooftop pool, where I find a spot to float in the steaming water on my own, contemplating the early evening mist as it curls itself around the rooftops and spires. The abbey bells are ringing as the sky drains of color. This is perfect. It *is* possible. I'll get there. I know I will.

I have a glass of wine in my dressing gown and then get dressed and go for a wander around the shops. My favorite boutiques are gone, swept aside by the new rules of the hyper-capitalist, hedge-fund nightmare that runs the British high street in 2014. I still need a new pair of sunglasses, so on a whim I go into Sunglass Hut. They have the most perfect pair of Prada mirrored aviators. They cost the same as one night in the posh spa hotel. I buy them, while "Ray Charles" by Chiddy Bang plays in the background. On the way home I download a couple of Chiddy Bang albums. This is the soundtrack that will carry me thought the rest of the year: music that is bright, irreverent, and punky-cheerful. All surface, no depth. Like me.

7

Sutton

The problem with being the hero of your own narrative is not just that you have to suffer, because that seems inevitable, but that you have to change. I am on a journey, but to where? I know I should probably discover that it's pointless trying to find meaning in tennis, or that winning isn't that good. But winning is fucking awesome and it's all I want to do. I don't want to change; I just want to win. If I do change I want the trajectory to be simple: zero to hero, nobody to champion. But it has not happened yet. I've won one tournament, and one further match, but I seem to be stalled, going nowhere.

•

I get back from Bath on Monday afternoon. On Tuesday, April 8, we celebrate Rod's birthday, which is actually the following day, by going to Sissinghurst and then to dinner, where we drink a lovely bottle of Margaux and talk about *Game of Thrones* and tennis. We've watched a couple of episodes of *Game of Thrones* and are uncertain about continuing. All that violence, all those breasts. But I like a lot of new things now. I used to be a timid vegetarian who was fond of cricket. Now I want the blood and guts of meat, rugby, tennis. Does tennis actually have blood and guts? Maybe.

We can't celebrate Rod's birthday on the proper day because I have to go to the Canongate London Book Fair dinner, where a little speech will be made about me and my upcoming book. It's important that I go: my foreign publishers will be there, and loads of people from Canongate. I can't believe that I also have to miss a tennis coaching session—the second this week. All I want to do is play tennis. But instead I have to get my hair done and then go and drink prosecco in a hot room full of people who secretly wish they were doing something else.

I've never worked out how to "do" these parties. At least I now have a theme: tennis always gives me something to talk about. So I start making jokes about how I should have a play-off with Geoff Dyer to see who should write Canongate's tennis book until someone reminds me he's just had a stroke. People ask me what my new book is about and I say it's about how evil plants really are, and how they make us do what they want, and then my ex-agent, Simon, walks in and then I'm chatting to someone from a New York publisher that just rejected my book and some nice-looking kid keeps coming around and pouring more prosecco. He's tall and fit-looking. I wonder if, like me, he'd rather be playing tennis. An author friend of mine is drinking sparkling mineral water. He seems to begin every evening saying he's not going to drink and then ends up slaughtered anyway.

I hug Simon. We look at each other awkwardly. We used to be such good friends; now this.

"How's your dad?" Simon asks, out of the blue. People are watching our exchange. I'm sure no one knows our history or why this is so weird but they must be able to feel it. The atmosphere is like a pane of glass about to shatter. Why is he asking about my father?

"Wasn't he the manager of OMD or something? And then didn't he get sacked by Virgin Records and go off and work as a bloodstock agent?"

Simon then bombards me with every fact about my life that he knows. He asks me about my ex, the one I left for Rod. How *is* he? What's he doing now? The sad thing is that I know Simon's not doing this on purpose to hurt me back. He's just nervous, saying the things coming into his mind. At least, I hope that's the explanation. It's extremely odd. But then how is he supposed to know that almost every aspect of my life, everything he could pull out of my past, is painful?

After that I go and stand in an empty room upstairs for a while.

Over dinner I learn that friends of the film director sitting on my right moved to California so their daughter could play tennis there. We talk about *Infinite Jest*. I tell them some anecdotes from various tennis books. I don't talk about my novel or their films—too obvious. Jamie Byng gets up and talks about my "beautiful book" that isn't actually out until the following year. I leave early to get the last train from St. Pancras but then sit in it for two and a half hours while police chase some kids out of the tunnel just beyond Stratford. "Just run the little cunts over," the people across the aisle from me are saying. I sit quietly reading my John McEnroe book, drunk enough to be pretty fine with what's happening, but—thank God—not so drunk I can't read at all.

The next day is Thursday. I'm hungover. I finally got home at around 3:30 a.m. I haven't played tennis all week. I am still reliving the humiliation of the Bath tournament in my head, although this is starting to resolve from "I'm a dick because I lost" into "Next time I will win." If those girls can do it, there's no reason why I can't. They have coaching; I have coaching. It's as simple as that. Though I won't be able to take it if Dan covers my racquet with a carrier bag today to try to teach me topspin, or constructs a "washing line" for me to hit over. I don't think I can take any more humiliation.

Almost as if he knows exactly how I'm feeling, Dan bounces out of the office carrying his mini Bose speaker system. There's no one else in the tennis center, so we put music on and play along to it. His playlist is all recent hits like "Trumpets" by Jason Derulo and "Rather Be" by Clean Bandit. This is exactly the right music to play tennis to. At one point I connect my iPhone to the speaker, but my playlist—the same one I've had since Leicester—feels timeworn and melancholy and not at all motivational, so we go back to Dan's music.

Our one-hour session has begun at 2:00 p.m. "Shall we go until half four?" Dan asks me nonchalantly when we stop for a drink. I immediately text the person I was due to have afternoon tea with and cancel. It's amazing. The music shoots me right into the zone and holds me there. I am no longer tired or hungover. We hardly stop, going through basket after basket of balls, hitting rallies that are both competitive and cooperative. We want to keep them going, but we also want to win them. This is my very favorite sort of tennis. I feel myself dropping into a super-relaxed focus. I know I can hit a basic forehand now, wherever I want on the court. So what happens if I brush the top of the ball more? What happens if I try this combination of shots? None of this is exactly Self 1 stuff, though. It feels like Self 2—my higher, chilled self—is having a wonderful playtime. For the whole session I don't care about anything other than hitting the ball, getting it back one more time, curious about how I hit it and where it goes without being judgmental. By the time I get home all I can do is collapse into a bath.

I come back for more the following day, but there are people around and Dan and I have to go off to Court 4 and only have the music on quietly down at one end. This becomes the "music end" and we entertain each other by dancing each time we arrive there, to music that the other cannot hear. Today we play points. It's not like last week when I almost beat him. This week feels more like business as usual. I'm in the wrong place on the court as another winner rips past me. What is the difference between last week and this week? How did I do that, instead of this? Or is it just that Dan is playing a lot better?

I'm a little distracted because this season's teams are being pinned up on the wall. Afterward I go and look at them. There are the two mixed teams, both of which I agreed to play on and captain and . . . oh. I'm not actually on the team for the East Kent league. A weaker woman than me is there instead. WTF? I sigh, wondering how to bring this up with Margaret. Surely she remembers the conversation we had where I said I didn't want to play ladies' doubles and she asked if I wanted to be on both mixed teams? But I imagine she hasn't remembered, that once again, a commitment I thought I'd made just never really existed.

That weekend we have Rod's daughter Daisy, her husband Ed, and their three children to stay. I spend Saturday holding Eliza, seven, upside-down and playing football with her. I'm feeling energized and excited: on Sunday I have my first Aegon match. Before I leave on Sunday morning Molly, who is eight, tells me earnestly that it doesn't matter whether I win or lose; it's how I play that counts. Eliza simply says, "WIN WIN WIN WIN WIN."

When I arrive at the leisure center, much too early because I wanted to free up the shower for the guests at home, I make the big mistake of walking past the desk because the queue is too long. But it's the grumpy receptionist Dolly, and she phones down to the gym to say I never waited to get my card swiped, so I get told off just before I'm meant to play. Brilliant. Then Lyn in the café refuses to put my stuff for afternoon tea in the fridge. I do wonder why on earth I am playing tennis for this place. But it turns out that today I'm not. The opposition simply never shows up.

We play doubles anyway, Margaret and me against Sara and Helen, both fill-ins brought in at the last minute. Helen is a solid second-team player and Sara is a rich chick from Sandwich with her own tennis court and—I think—a nice splash of Dior's Bois d'Argent. She smells lovely. She is lovely. She has a nice hard topspin forehand, a lot of gold jewelry, and a body that looks like it knows how to have fun. I like her immediately. I suspect we share a personal trainer—mine talked about training a woman in Sandwich with her own tennis court.

Sara and Helen are solid players, but they should not win the first set from Margaret and me. They do, 6–4. We win the next one 7–5, but still. When I get home I commission Eliza to draw me a picture of me winning a tennis match. I have to mentally prepare for the Sutton Tennis Academy Easter Grade 2 Tournament, which I have entered on the basis that the ladies' singles is Grade 3 and I already see that some 9.1s and 9.2s have entered. Eliza's picture is dominated by a gray net running across the middle of the page. On one side of this net, at the bottom of the page, is a thin girl with brown hair and a purple smile, dressed in purple, with a trophy and the word WINER. But the girl at the top of the page stands out more. She has a green and orange outfit and purple hair. Her green lips are curled down in a sad face. LOOSER! it says at the top. I know, deep down, that this is me.

•

I've been reading a new book on mindfulness and eating. I can't stop wondering about why exactly I remain the same weight no matter how much exercise I do. I've noticed that I seem unable to go to tennis without a bottle of Lucozade that contains roughly the same number of calories I'll be burning off, and of course when I've been exercising I give myself permission to eat more.

But it's not even as simple as that. I think some unconscious part of me wants to remain the same size and I don't know why. If I know I'm playing tennis later, I sort of panic and pile on the calories because I believe they are fuel, and I might get tired without them. Can I blame my mother for this? Probably. She has that metabolism that burns everything up and constantly needs food. If she doesn't get her lunch on the dot of midday (or preferably 11:45), she becomes homicidal.

I have also begun realizing the extent to which I emotionally eat, and that is what this new book is about. Instead of eating the numbing, quick-fix piece of chocolate or toast, it suggests, you could try experiencing your actual feelings instead. This immediately makes sense to me. I hadn't realized the extent to which I now eat the way I used to smoke. Bad feeling? Light up—although these days it's the fridge that lights up, rather than the cigarette. Of course I never exactly overdo it. I've never been much of a binge eater, unless you count having three pieces of toast instead of two, or just a bit more than a normal portion of cheese with my soup.

But it all adds up. The bits of Green & Black's chocolate bars I sneak from the cupboard while the kettle boils. The extra butter I add to everything. My feeling that I need food: that without it I might die, or at the very least feel a bit hard done by. Rod and I agree that I am the better cook, but I'm not sure he knows this is because I am the freest with the ingredients. Everything I make comes with cream, olive oil, or butter. I buy big steaks when he would buy small ones, two packets of king prawns when he would buy one. It's not that I don't try. I periodically cut things out, but when I don't have dairy I just have more olive oil. I give up wheat but spend whole days eating gluten-free toast. It's just so frustrating. Like my forehand, like my career, like everything in my life: my weight seems stuck.

•

Going away to a tennis tournament means eating and drinking what I like. After all, I'm staying in a hotel—the Croydon Hilton—and this is like a holiday. Remember: nothing you do in a hotel counts. None of it is normal life. Still, I limit myself to one gin and tonic on the Tuesday night before my first match. But I also eat a big steak and chips and have a pudding. The pudding is deemed "healthy" by Hilton. It is a bowl full of strawberries covered in a kind of mint syrup with a huge portion of thick cream on the top. Even I leave half the cream.

Somewhere at the back of my mind I am aware that I have over one thousand emails, at least four hundred of them unread. I am a week late with a book review. Radio 3 just got in touch to ask if I'd like to do a piece for them on a garden Kipling liked. It's to be recorded on July 3. There's an LTA tournament in Spain then that I have tentatively signed up for, but even if I am not in Spain I'll certainly be doing something tennis related, during the second week of Wimbledon and two days before my birthday. So I turn it down.

I have stopped opening letters. I have not taken my car in for its service. I still have piles of research from two books ago that I have not put away. But who cares, right? Especially at this moment, when I am more or less On Holiday. Do I deserve a holiday? No, not really. OK, then. This is *work*. I am writing my very important tennis book and that is why I am here. I don't convince myself. At this moment tennis feels like video games used to, when I would spend six hours at a time engaged only with the pixels on the TV, trying desperately to win but not sure why, shoring up weapons and lives and skills against an uncertain, violent future.

Still, here I am. The Croydon Hilton is cheerful. When I checked in, the receptionist asked if I was a professional tennis player. I almost feel like one as I prepare for my first match in the Sutton Tennis Academy Easter Grade 2 Tournament tomorrow morning. It feels like a miracle that I'm actually here. In the last few weeks, almost every tournament I've signed up for has not run due to lack of interest. It's like a large, complicated game all its own. You can see people signing up and leaving. I'm even starting to recognize some of the players' names: people from Leicester, from the Spring Open. Siobhan Clarke has signed up for Sutton, and a couple of other women with a similar profile to me, but it's always a bit knife-edge and strategic. No one wants to end up in a tournament in which only three other people are playing. No one wants to be the highest-rated player in a tournament (well, unless they are sure they can win it) because no one wants qualifying losses. In order to go up to an 8.1, which will prove to Margaret that I was right to start at 8.2, I need three qualifying wins this season. I'm not off to a good start. A qualifying win is against a player of the same rating or higher. What you can't do is lose to anyone rated lower than you. So far I've beaten an 8.2, lost to an 8.2, and lost to a 4.1 and a 5.2. If I can win a couple of matches here, I'm bound to go up.

How likely is that? While I am engaged in my pre-tournament ritual of watching Rafa clips on YouTube, an email comes through from the tournament organizers. I am to go to lta.tournamentsoftware. com to check my start time, which has now been published. I have

assumed that it's going to be 8:30 but am thrilled to see it's actually
9:30, which means an extra hour in bed. Or just more time to worry.
But how worried am I really? I can see that I'm playing a 9.2. Charanya was a 9.2, and although I played timidly against her in Leicester
and allowed her three games, I think I'd blast her now. I love lta.
tournamentsoftware.com. It's the online equivalent of backstage at
a tennis event. You can see draws, timings, surfaces. Although no
surface has yet been assigned to the women's singles, I can see from
the draw diagram that if I do beat Rachel MacDonald at 9:30, then
at 12:30 I'll be playing the top seed Helen Clements, a nineteen-year-
old 4.1 from Sussex. Obviously she'll thrash me. Fine. Then I'll come
back to the hotel and drink red wine. It's a plan. I sleep well, dreaming
of tennis as usual.

The next morning is bright and sunny. My minicab takes me
through endless suburbs. I hadn't realized quite how far my hotel
is from Sutton, quite how much stuff there really is before South
London turns into Gatwick. We go past duck ponds in faux village
greens. Hawthorn is blossoming, daffodils line the roads. Everything is a detached house, a park, or a garden. The sun is shining. It's
going to be a hot day, apparently. The first real warmth of the year.

I am the first person to sign in for the ladies' singles at 8:40. I
was hoping to find Siobhan Clarke so we could knock up before our
first matches. She's still an 8.2, like me, and her position on the other
side of the draw almost exactly mirrors mine. She's playing a 9.1,
Alexandra Groszek. If she beats her she gets to play the second seed,
Olivia Parson. I haven't seen Siobhan since the Spring Open, but I'm
sure we've both noticed that we've been entering some of the same
tournaments. Given that hardly anyone enters these tournaments,
it's clear we have something unusual in common: we are both over
thirty and we have both been bitten by the tournament bug. I wish

I'd beaten her at the Indoor Tennis Centre. I should have beaten her then. But there are no hard feelings and I must admit I'd quite like to see a familiar face at this moment.

This is by far the most well-organized tournament I have played in. The kids' matches are all Grade 2 and the semifinals and finals actually have real umpires sitting up on high plastic chairs calling balls in and out and keeping track of the score. There seem to be a lot of clay courts and some acrylic courts. I'm half-hoping to get my first go on clay, although I realize that would be mad, as I've never played on it before. When I ask the organizer, he's not sure, but he says it probably will be clay. I admit it: I am excited.

Each match is called over a loudspeaker. After you hear your name called, you have to go to the desk to find out what court you've been allocated. A man comes with you and flips a coin, then times a five-minute warm-up. Officials walk around in case there's any dispute. I bump into Siobhan just before my match is called. She's been stuck in traffic but would have loved a hit. We wish each other luck and agree to catch up later.

My opponent, Rachel MacDonald, is a nice Scottish woman in her early thirties. We are assigned Court 23, which is clay. I gulp. It's not quite the sticky red earth I imagined—it's actually kind of powdery. When we start hitting, I'm surprised to encounter a topspin forehand more like Lucille's than Charanya's. She hits it hard and deep. Oh crap. Am I going to lose *again*? I win the toss and decide to receive. And then it turns out that Rachel is extremely nervous, or has the yips on her serve, or something. Her ground strokes are great but she serves two double faults in the first game, which I take easily. The scoreboard has our names chalked on it and we have been instructed that we must keep it updated on the changeovers. 1–0 to me. It's a start. I struggle a bit to find rhythm with my first service game and it goes to deuce, but I do win it. Then I win her service game. At the next changeover it's 3–0. *OMG*, I think, *she's really good but I'm actually going to win this.* I might even win it 6–0, 6–0. I imagine telling Rod. Telling Dan. Going back to the leisure center with a double bagel in an actual Grade 3 tournament.

Rachel wins the next game. And the next three after that. I realize only when I think about it later that she has been hitting her shots freely, and even though quite a lot of them have sailed out early on, she has now found the lines. I have been playing more carefully, building an advantage out of her mistakes. But now she's making fewer mistakes and I'm stuck with my hesitant comfort-play. Her serve is still terrible, though, and I break it again for 4–4, but I'm not hitting enough winners and I don't really have any kind of game plan beyond seeing what she does and responding as best I can. I don't really know how to play on clay. It looks good on TV but it's kind of slippery. I see now why the players do that slidey thing, but I can't do it. Rachel sends me wide on the backhand and then blasts a winner down my forehand side. On acrylic I might have been able to recover and get to the shot. On clay? Not a chance.

But we both want to win this. I come into the net a few times, but again get more points off the errors forced by the surprise factor than off playing actual winners myself. The clay is heavy but also dusty, and you have to "sweep the lines," with an actual broom, after playing on it. In fact, the lines could do with a sweep now. I can't see the baseline. I can't see the inner tramline on the deuce side. My brain needs to see the lines in order to be able to hit them. I send balls deep into what I think is the far deuce court corner. "Out," calls Rachel. It's 5–5. If I can get the next game and serve for the set ... but I don't get it, and Rachel gets the set 7–5. Fuck. I've gone from 3–0 up to 7–5 down. How did that happen? I feel like crying.

It is very warm, and I'm wearing my tennis skirt without leggings underneath for the first time ever. I began feeling free because of this, but in fact my thighs are rubbing together and chafing. Not only does this hurt, it's confirmation that I am fat.

I am a fat loser, I think, going into the second set.

Rachel never quite gets her serve together, but her attacking ground strokes get better and better. I do keep playing in the second set, but she plays better than me and takes it 6–4. When we shake hands at the net I tell her this is the first time I've played on clay. I'm hoping that she'll admit to being a clay expert, which will give me the excuse I need for this. But no, she's only played on clay on holiday, and that was real clay, not this artificial stuff. This clay is artificial? I guess it is.

We go back to the tournament desk to give our result. I feel fucking awful. There is literally no joy in this. I'm told that players have fifteen minutes to sign up for the consolation event after losing their first match. I still can't believe I *have* lost my first match. I feel like I need a lot more than fifteen minutes to process it. Siobhan is sitting at a table with a blonde woman in a yellow Stella McCartney top, whom she introduces as Stela Krumova. I wonder if she's her next opponent.

"How did you do?" Siobhan asks me.

I make a face and shake my head. "You?"

"I won!" she says. "I can't believe it. I lost the first set 6–0, won the next one 6–1, and then scraped through the tiebreak 11–9."

"Well done," I say, trying to sound like I mean it. Do I wish she'd lost? Of course I do. I'm human. Also: How does someone lose a first set 6–0 and then win the next one 6–1? It's too weird.

I take a consolation draw form from the desk. Hope starts to trickle through me again. I couldn't possibly lose twice, could I? I assume these matches will be played today, but when I ask the organizer he says that they'll begin tomorrow. Crap. Do I really want to go through another whole day of this? I have no hotel booked tomorrow night, so I'd have to check out tomorrow morning and bring my suitcase here. It's way too much hassle. I put the form back. I could go home now. But then what about my red wine? It's Wednesday night, which is a non-drinking night at home, but if I remain On Holiday then I can drink as much as I like. Then again, if I'm playing the consolation draw I'd better not drink too much. Although that approach hasn't helped me today. I could pretend I'm playing in the McEnroe era and come tomorrow with a hangover and see if that helps.

I go out and sit on the grass in the sunshine and text my result to Dan. Then I ring Rod. He's lovely. A match doesn't get much closer than 7–5, 6–4, although perhaps Siobhan's freakish result is mathematically closer. Of course, I should have taken it to three sets. I should have won the second set and then lost the tiebreak. Or maybe even won the tiebreak! But I hate tiebreaks. I tell him how strange it was playing on clay, but also how I somehow didn't want to win, can't have wanted to win. How could I throw away a 3–0 lead? He thinks I should stay on and play the consolation draw. Get some more practice on clay. I must admit that playing outside in the sun is lovely, even with the chafing. Right now I don't want to leave this place, where it feels properly warm for the first time this year, and where there is nothing in the world apart from tennis. I've come all the way here. I should play more than one match.

It turns out that Stela is Siobhan's friend from the Dartford David Lloyd Tennis Centre. Stela is playing next, so I go with Siobhan to the grassy hill behind the far clay courts to watch her. Two courts over, Rachel is playing Helen Clements in the match I hoped I was going to be playing, so we watch that at the same time. I half-hope Rachel wins, because if the person who knocked me out also knocks out the top seed then that makes a good story. But I also hope she loses because she beat me and I want her to suffer. But she's certainly playing well and the rallies are a lot longer than the ones I had with Vanessa Brill.

"There's no way she's a 9.2," says Siobhan.

"I know," I say.

"The girl I played wasn't a 9.1 either. No way."

"At least you beat her."

"Yeah." Siobhan chuckles. "I was amazed."

"How exactly did you turn it around from 6–0?"

"Took the pace off the ball. She likes to hit it hard so I just took all the pace off." She laughs again. I smile. It's the same tactic she used on me in the ITC.

On the clay court below us, Stela is floundering. Apparently Stela has recently gone up from an 8.1 to a 7.2. She's playing a 7.1. Siobhan tells me that Stela hits with her husband every day, that she's obsessed with tennis. But then that's true of all of us here. I learn that Siobhan's partner is a tennis coach. I assume, although don't ask, that both Siobhan and Stela don't have children. Like me.

I suddenly get a warm glow. Here I am with women I have things in common with—not a love of literature or an understanding of phenomenology or an interest in contemporary art—other things. Earthier things. In John McEnroe's book there is a real sense of what it was like going around tournaments in the '70s and '80s, bumping into friends and rivals and just deciding on the spur of the moment to enter the doubles with some pal you've run into in the locker room, or the bar. At John McEnroe's first Wimbledon he ended up entering the mixed doubles on a whim with his childhood friend Mary Carillo. In this spirit I ask Siobhan if she'd like to enter the doubles with me, but she has to get home.

I yawn, stretch back onto the grass. The sun is lovely. Even though I feel like a loser, it's nice here with the sounds of tennis all around me. Planes fly over. There are a few bees. Siobhan gets out some sunscreen. I realize that even though my tennis bag contains, among other things, four types of bandage, three types of painkiller, lipstick, spare change, extra fluid, liquid chalk, various changes of clothes, and three tennis racquets, I do not have sunscreen. Siobhan offers me some of hers. I put a bit on my ankles, but really, how harsh can the sun be in England in April?

Rachel finishes playing. It didn't look like she was losing heavily—and Siobhan thought maybe she was even winning—but her score is 6–2, 6–1. It is a heavy loss, but for a 9.2 against a 4.1 it's actually pretty good. Stela comes off and joins us. She has lost more badly: 6–1, 6–0. She blames the clay, and a pain in her side, and flops down next to us. She's wearing cool earrings with her bright yellow top. She has sharp cheekbones and insouciant, slutty-in-a-good-way makeup. I really like her. She's going to be in the consolation draw with me. If there is an in-crowd at this tournament, I suddenly realize, we are it. When Rachel comes over to us we are possibly a little cold with her. She drifts away. Siobhan starts speculating about whether or not Stela and I will play each other. On the court below us, Rushan Tonge-Bobia, the big-haired Black girl who I last saw at Leicester, is being beaten by the third seed. "I bet you'll actually end up playing her," Siobhan says to Stela. For me she predicts Alexandra Groszek. She's right both times.

There's no gluten-free food here so I get a cup of tea instead. Stela and I watch Siobhan get double-bagelled by the second seed. I keep checking my phone for a reply from Dan, but nothing comes.

Afterward, Siobhan is keen to get home. Stela's second match is also tomorrow, like mine. She's going to drive home and then come back, but she's not in such a hurry.

"Do you fancy a hit?" she asks me.

"What, now?"

"Sure. There're lots of free courts."

She's right. It's approaching 4:00 p.m. and most of the matches are over. There's an early summer, early evening feel to the place. We go down to the courts and start hitting. Stela is a surprisingly competitive hitter, more determined to win points than keep the rally going. But it's OK. It's just nice to get some more practice on the clay.

A family turns up on the next court. A big woman in a floral skirt, two children, and a dog. The little boy starts running around with the dog. The woman has a large carrier bag with her. It is full of mangled-looking tennis balls. The little girl goes to one side of the net, and the mother starts feeding balls to her.

"Hit it!" she shouts, her voice heavily accented. "Move yourrrrr feet!"

This is the soundtrack to the rest of my hit with Stela. The mother shouts at her daughter frequently in English but also in some other language.

"Move! Lazy! *Hit it!*"

"It's Bulgarian," says Stela, when we break for a drink.

"What's she saying?" I ask.

Stela laughs. "Stuff like the daughter is useless, worthless."

"Fuck."

"Yeah. Right now she's threatening to beat her with the tennis racquet."

•

I've finished the McEnroe book, and so my companion on this trip is Serena Williams's *My Life*. What is it about tennis parents? Serena's father Richard apparently drew up a seventy-eight-page plan for his daughters' tennis careers when Serena was around four years old. He was listed in the "pushy fathers" speech in the "Teddy Perkins" episode of *Atlanta*, which I now use to teach students the Gothic. I read all about how Richard Williams ordered instructional videos and books and tried out their techniques on his wife, then pregnant with Venus, while I eat my large dinner, after my long bath and massive gin and tonic. Some years later I'll be having dinner with a poet who's come to examine one of my PhD students, and he will laughingly, sheepishly, admit to a tennis-parent episode of his own that culminated in him writing to the LTA to ask them to ban another parent—previously a close friend—from coming within ten feet of his son.

Right now, I am exhausted and sunburnt. My chafing has left red welts on my inner thighs. But I can carry on, right? Surely, surely I can't lose again tomorrow? I picture myself beating Alexandra Groszek and then patiently working my way through the rest of the consolation draw. It could happen. I need to win more than ever now, because my loss against Rachel MacDonald has neutralized my win against Sharon. I need three new qualifying wins to go up to an 8.1. Or maybe four, actually, since I think we're in a new season now.

The next day I get my cab driver to stop at a drugstore and I buy Piz Buin sunscreen and some Vaseline to rub on my thighs. Nothing is going to stop me. At Sutton Tennis Academy it's clearly boy day. There are under-14, under-16, and under-18 matches going on everywhere. It's hard to see where the women's consolation draw is going to fit in. When I arrive, two under-16s are really going at it on Court 18. One of them cries when a ball he thought was in was called out by his opponent. He goes all the way to the opposite baseline to examine the mark—clay encourages this kind of drama—but there is no mark. The other boy loses the set and then he cries too. For the rest of the match they shout things at each other. "So late!" yells one of them after his serve is called out only after the other boy has fluffed his return. "Just because your shot was so lame." There are tennis parents everywhere. One dad complains to another that his son doesn't like the courts wet, but doesn't like them dry either. I overhear a mother on her phone telling her husband how well their son is hitting the ball today, despite "significant pressure on his backhand."

Sometimes contemplating pro tennis is like contemplating the entire universe, or at least how many times you'd have to fold a piece of paper before it would reach to the moon. How many of these kids are going to make it? If "making it" means breaking into the top 250 in the world, say, then somewhere between one and none. Probably none. When he was this age, Andy Murray was in Spain playing against Rafa, not competing in bland LTA tournaments. Venus and Serena didn't do junior tournaments because even someone as bonkers as their father realized that they break people's spirits. Other big players who did play on junior circuits were so good that it's unlikely that any of them—even McEnroe—cried over line calls. Rafa was already winning under-12s easily at the age of eight. Then again, there is that story in his autobiography about the time he chose to have fun one summer rather than practice tennis and then lost a tournament. "I never want to feel like this again," he said to his father. Or something like that.

I feel like that too, after being beaten by Alexandra Groszek.

What happened during our match? I don't know. The score is recorded, but I didn't make any notes. The record tells a story of its own. The match took place on clay Court 21 and she won: 7–6 [3], 6–1. The three in brackets means that the set went to a tiebreak at 6–6 and that she won it 7–3. The score in the second set shows that I more or less gave up. I gave up, lost, and then what? Got my bag from where I'd left it behind the desk at reception and got in a cab and went to Sutton station and then to St. Pancras, where I probably bought another fluorescent sports bra from JD Sports, which used to be by the escalators up to Platforms 11, 12, and 13. But I actually have no idea what happened, because I made no notes. Between April 15 and 17, I also took no photographs (unthinkable now, as I write this in 2019, in a new age of limitless selfies and my Instagram Story to keep up). I'm sure I cried. I remember her being mean in some way, possibly a bit arsey. Was she maybe Polish? I remember vaguely wanting to say something about how my ex had been Polish. I think I wanted to be friendly, and she didn't.

Meanwhile, Stela was being beaten by Rushan Tonge-Bobia on clay Court 19. I don't remember whether we spoke again or not. We must have. Or maybe not. We started at the same time, and her match took one hour and fifty-five minutes, and mine took one hour and fifty. Maybe I simply used those five minutes to slip away because I couldn't bear to say anything or write anything or think anything about the fact that I'd lost yet again. Dan never responded to my message with my result from my first game, so I probably didn't even bother to send him another one. It's as if the whole thing never happened.

•

The following weekend, my brother Hari and his girlfriend Nia come to stay. They are such a lovely couple, beautiful, laid-back, and cool, but Hari is as competitive as I am, maybe more so. He's rarely played tennis. I think he had the odd knockabout in the park with Couze, but after Couze was diagnosed with angina in 1992, he became afraid of exercise and so didn't play so much sport. Hari was more of a football kid anyway, and a skateboarder. But he wants to play tennis now. He has the same gene as I do—that must come down my mother's line. The gene says *You can do anything you want.* It says *Miracles happen.* It says *There's always a chance the other person will die and you'll win by default.* Or, maybe (miracle!) you'll realize that you are a glorious undiscovered talent in ice-skating/ballet/tennis/whatever. Of course, if the miracle doesn't happen, there's no need to go back after that first session. No need to actually try, because trying is for losers and the uncool.

Hari therefore wonders whether he's been blessed with some incredible inner skill, undetected up until now, that means he will be able to thrash me, despite the fact that I train several times a week. Who knows? He could be right.

We go to the leisure center. The ITC is eerily empty. It's a good thing, because I don't look great playing Hari. He's naturally athletic and cool, but he stands out badly as an amateur in here. He hits the ball in high loops in the air. He does underspin. He has no follow-through. No backhand. No serve. I look good when I am playing a tennis professional who generates all the power. I can then whack the ball back and it looks like I have the same amount of power. During this session I realize how lame I truly am. Playing with Hari, I should look like a tennis professional myself. I should be able to deliver well-paced balls to his forehand that will make both of us look good. I can do this sometimes, but it's erratic. I'm basically shit.

While we are dibbly-dobblying the ball around, the green doors squeak open and some young guys come in. Are they Josh's friends? They go to Court 2 and start thwacking the ball around with power and verve. Then—oh God—Dan comes in with a woman I've never seen before. He waves at me, slightly embarrassed, and they go off to Court 4. I carry on looking like a bad recreational player who has never won a match in her life. Hari suggests we play some points. I give him three serves. It's fun, and he goes for every single point, but I do still beat him 6–0, 6–0.

"I see why you're doing this," he says afterward. "You're genuinely good."

But I'm not. Not really. And my arm hurts.

•

Tuesday. I am very worried about my arm, but excited about playing tennis today. Dan will be back at his Level 4 course for the rest of the week, so I won't have my Wednesday session. And then I leave with Rod for Venice on Sunday, which means I'll miss both my sessions next week. Dan never did respond to my text message with my first match result from Sutton, so I'm looking forward to talking to him about what went wrong. What can I work on now? More than anything, I want a confidence boost. I want to be able to hit the ball hard again. I want Dan to say something nice to me, to somehow make it all OK.

My pre-tennis routine is getting longer all the time. It starts properly when I wake up. If I'm playing tennis, that's usually my first thought of the day. Then I start counting down to the time I'm going to start. I think about what I can eat and drink to help me prepare. I have a little fizz in my stomach—part nerves, part excitement—that gets more intense as the day goes on. About an hour and a half before the official start of my session, I stop what I'm doing and begin getting ready. I get changed into my kit, pack my bag with a clean towel, my purse, my phone, and check the rest of my stuff is there: my three Juice racquets, my sweatbands, my spare top. Then I go downstairs to mix up my drink. Today it's Evian with green tea and nettle cordial. I am trying to make my own drinks fresh like this in the hope of stopping drinking Lucozade. And I'm also trying to increase the nutrient value of everything I consume, which means green tea rather than black tea and coconut oil rather than butter and so on. I am missing my big caffeine hits, though, and I feel oddly tearful.

I get to the leisure center early with the idea of spending a good amount of time warming up in the gym. But the nice girl behind the desk can't find my booking on the system.

"It's a private lesson," I say. "Dan should have put it on there."

"I can't see it," she says. "And the courts are all booked up for a tournament until four." She looks worried. She tries to phone the tennis office but gets no reply, so she sends me down. The place is unusually full of color and sound: kids, parents, mini-tennis balls, nets, and what seem like thousands of people with clipboards. Dan, Josh, and Margaret are there officiating the whole thing. Dan sees me and bounces over, sort of grimacing, but quite cheerful.

"Sorry!" he says. "I think it'll be over by three. Can we start then?"

Fine. I go to Sainsbury's and then to Walmer Tennis Club, looking for membership forms. Apparently everyone plays here in the summer. I've learned that it's usual for serious tennis players to be members of all the local clubs at once: the leisure center for when it rains, Canterbury for the clay and the good level of play, Walmer for perfectly manicured grass courts and the rule that everyone has to wear all white. I find Walmer's wrought iron gates dusty and pad-locked, like the beginning of a fairy tale, or perhaps a bit of a video game that you are not supposed to have found yet. The year 1886 is inscribed on the gates.

I get back to the leisure center around half past two so I can still do my warm-up in the gym. This time grumpy Dolly is at the desk too. I've already paid for my lesson, and the nice girl that gave me my receipt wants to wave me through, but I'm scared of getting into trouble so I make her sign me in for the gym, even though she obviously thinks this is unnecessary.

"Well, I hope you're not expecting to play tennis," Dolly says to me.

The other girl looks embarrassed. "She's got a lesson," she says to Dolly. "It's all arranged."

"Well, all I know is that all the courts are booked until four," says Dolly.

"She's arranged it directly with Dan," says the girl.

"Oh, I see. Got a hotline to the tennis coaches, have you?"

"I know how to send a text message," I say, a bit crisply.

When I go down to the tennis center at five past three, it's still chaos. Karen Bayliss is there, watching her son Daniel. None of the kids' matches look anywhere near ending.

"You're not expecting to have a tennis lesson in this chaos, are you?" Karen says.

"I'm sure it'll be fine."

But then Dan comes over and says that the tournament actually does go on until four, not three, and then he has to coach Daniel Bayliss as part of his course assessment, so we can't play at all today. He offers me Saturday afternoon, but I'll be on my way to Gatwick then. I'm becoming unhappy. Is he incapable of texting me to let me know what's going on? I have a block booking for Tuesday after-noon. No one told me it was canceled today. I don't say anything for a few seconds. I'm sort of stunned.

"Can I at least use the ball machine?" I ask. I can see Court 4 is free.

"The thing is the schools have booked all the courts and paid for them until four," he says. "So probably not. Hang on. I'll check."

But then a parent comes and asks him for a bandage and I can see he's swamped in this tournament. He makes a kind of "sorry" face at me, and I actually make a kind of "fuck you" face back. I mean, this is just stupid. I am already crying as I leave the leisure center, hoping Dolly can't see me. I feel like a child. I drive to the seafront and sob my heart out because my tennis coaching session was canceled. OK, not just that, but because no one told me. And then Daniel got a spare slot and I didn't. And Daniel is an up-and-coming kid and I'm just a pathetic old woman with a hollow dream. That thing Dan said to his Level 4 instructor about a "lady" at his club having the same Juice racquet as him comes back to me. That time he called me a recreational player. He thinks I am a joke. I am being coached by someone who thinks I am a joke, who doesn't even bother to tell me that my session is canceled. I have a book review due tomorrow. I got up at 6:00 a.m. to work on it so I could play ten-nis at 2:30 with a clear conscience. Does Dan not think I have a life?

Maybe he's right. I feel like a fucking loser.

When I get home I wonder about giving tennis a rest for a few days. We leave for Venice on Saturday. My arm hurts a lot, although I've actually hardly played tennis for the last week. There was just that session with Hari. But, still, maybe I should rest it some more? Then again, if I rested everything that hurt I'd never play tennis again. I sent a message to Luke, but haven't heard back, which I

208 • SCARLETT THOMAS

assume means he's not going to be around on Thursday. I have two hours with Lee on Wednesday. Perhaps I should cancel that too and just have a good period of time off.

Or I could text Margaret and ask if Josh is available.

I've avoided doing this since last time, as I sensed there was some problem. Had I broken some rule of etiquette by having a buddy hit with Josh when Dan is officially my coach? But fuck it. Now I have nothing to lose. I text Margaret and say that as my two sessions with Dan have been canceled this week, does Josh have any slots free? The next morning I get a text from Josh himself. Yes, he's around. When do I want to play? We arrange two sessions: one for Wednesday at 2:00 p.m. and another for Friday at 4:00. There are matches going on that should finish by 2:00, but Josh says he'll text me by 1:40 just to confirm. He doesn't, he says, want a repeat of the "disaster" of yesterday.

So they did realize.

•

When I arrive at the leisure center, there are two people behind the desk: Dolly and the nice girl from the other day. But the nice girl is on the phone. At least there's no queue today.

"Hello, Scarlett," says Dolly cheerfully, in her low, treacly, northern voice.

Perhaps I could try neutralizing her again?

"Hi, Dolly," I say. "How are you?"

"So busy," she says, sighing.

"Is it still Easter?" I say. "Or have the kids gone back now?"

"They've gone back. But we're still *so* busy."

"OK, well, can I have a buddy hit with Josh please, beginning at 2:00 p.m.?"

This is simple. And it is five to two so she can't tell me I'm here too early or have a go at me for not officially signing into the gym or taking my bag in there or whatever because I'm not even going to the gym. I have my membership card and my business debit card ready. Nothing can go wrong.

"Spend all your pocket money on tennis lessons, don't you?" she says.

I try to smile politely. "Something like that."

"I mean," she goes on, "you don't pay my entire wages but you must come quite close."

Ouch. How does she do this? She's like a pro tennis player who can hit a winner from anywhere on the court. Even though I have not done anything wrong, she has found a way to get to me. Why?

•

Last time I hit with Josh, he said he didn't want to interfere with what Dan was doing with me. "Treat me like a ball machine," he said. Today, after we've been hitting for ten minutes or so, he comes to the net.

"I don't want to interfere with what Dan is doing with you," he says, "but . . ."

"Go on, interfere," I say.

He starts instructing me on my forehand. It's not as if poor Dan hasn't been hammering away at my forehand for months now, but Josh just says one or two key things and they work. Am I like one of those puppies that won't sit for its master but will do it for guests? Then again, sometimes it works with Dan too, but then in a couple of sessions I go back to my old forehand and it feels comfortable and it works OK—but I'm not winning matches with it against any but the very wildest hitters. Josh also gives me a different grip: a full western.

"The thing is," he says, "that grip that Dan uses and that you've been using is a bit old-fashioned now."

Right. OK. Game on, it seems.

Still, one nice thing about Josh is that he gives feedback that isn't all bad.

"Good," he says. "Those last four were great. But the fifth one, did you feel how that was different? You were scooping again."

The only thing that bothers me a bit is that Dan only ever says pleasant, positive, admiring things about Josh, telling me stories about the holes Josh makes in balls because he whacks them so hard, and all the winners he hits when they play together. But Josh is not so nice about Dan.

"What does he actually do with you?" he asks me as we leave the court after our session is complete.

"Well, lately we've just been putting loud music on and whacking balls to each other," I say. I don't add that I love doing this almost more than anything in the world. I guess I'm still sore about Tuesday, and about losing the week before. The lack of responses to my texts. Did I lose because I practice to music rather than slavishly improving my forehand? At this moment that feels like as good an excuse as any.

Josh looks unimpressed.

"The thing is," he says, "while it's not always true that the best tennis players make the best coaches, in this case I think you could learn more from me. Especially given what you're trying to achieve."

"Could that work?" I say. "What's the etiquette of maybe having you as my actual coach and Dan as more of a hitting partner?"

Obviously I know the answer to this. In tennis terms it's like leaving your husband to shag someone else while hoping you can still "remain friends." Or like sacking your agent—and friend—of more than ten years. I am a bad person.

In my defense, I have to say that it is only Wednesday and I am still very cross about Tuesday. And Josh has just taught me loads about my forehand. But I still sort of hate myself. Dan is my friend. It's true that he sometimes doesn't reply to my messages, and our sessions often begin five minutes late. On the other hand, Josh's lessons finish on the dot while Dan's are likely to go on for an extra half hour, hour, or more. Josh so obviously plays down to me and says so. Today, after a particularly excruciating rally that left me gasping for a break and a drink, I said something like "Wow, what a tough point," and he said, "Yes, I just put the ball where I thought it would stretch you just the right amount."

Friday's session is exhilarating. Josh gets out a basket of the best Head Pro balls—my favorites—which he has clearly assembled beforehand. He feeds them to me and I hit forehand after forehand down the line. Winner after winner after winner. Of course, it helps that there's no one on the other side of the net. After this I'm dripping with sweat, developing that post-exercise high that some people say burns you out if you abuse it.

While we're having a drink, Josh asks me about my book. He seems genuinely interested—he is, after all, a grammar school boy with good manners.

"I don't think Dan reads very many books," he says.

"No," I agree.

"Right," says Josh, springing up from his chair. "Enough lazing about. I want to teach you a two-handed backhand. It's what you need."

"OK," I say. "Cool. Although . . ."

He grins at me like a kid caught mid-prank. "What?"

"Well, when I next play Dan. If I turn up with a two-handed backhand then he'll know."

"Fuck him," says Josh.

•

Home later, showered and foam-rolled. Rod's out at a New Zealand Studies Network thing. I've got a gin and tonic and some tennis to watch and I should feel happy but instead I feel flat. I just can't imagine going into the tennis center to train for neat clipped hours with Josh and not playing with Dan any more. Then again, I see Dan as a friend. How does he see me? Am I just some chick with a bit of money that he has to coach, or does he see me as a friend too? Tomorrow Rod and I are packing and leaving for a night at Gatwick before our early flight to Venice. No more tennis for me until I get back. This, too, makes me feel flat. I compose a text to Dan. I tell him I've had a couple of sessions with Josh and that I hope he doesn't mind but it was the only way I could get any tennis this week, as the person I hit with in Canterbury has a bad back. Would he be free maybe the Saturday or Sunday after I get back? I hit send and feel a little bit better about myself. Then I watch Rafa lose to Nicolas Almagro in the quarterfinals of Barcelona. Rafa isn't hitting it deep enough, with enough belief. It's hard to tell what's wrong with him. He's ahead for the whole match and then he loses.

8

The Canterbury Open

We are about to fly home from Venice. I've been eating wheat and I feel weird. It started a week ago with a little pastry from a shop just over a little bridge by where we were staying near St. Rocco. But it has ended with a full-on sandwich and pastry binge at the airport. OK, not a "binge" exactly: I don't do that. It's basically one and a half miniature pastries and three and a half little sandwiches with protein fillings. But I feel all wrong inside.

I've been avoiding gluten for the last few months because I seem to feel better when I do. But when we got to our hotel last week, it became clear that this was going to have to go on hold: breakfast was all freshly cooked bread and pastries. Even if there had been gluten-free bread, I wasn't going to have it. I'm not that crazy. For the first few days I felt OK, and wondered if my food intolerances—like everything else—are in my head. But now I feel wheated out: bloated, sleepy, grumpy. I'm the seven dwarfs all at once, or maybe the seven deadly sins.

Does it even matter?

Just this morning I stood in St. Rocco looking at Tintoretto's *Crucifixion* and I felt something important. For the first time ever

I properly understood that what Jesus is telling us is that the body doesn't matter. This life doesn't matter. Put yourself in the hands of the universe and get somewhere else. Get out of this place, with its inequalities, its cruelties, its winning and losing. On the way up the stairs in St. Rocco I slightly strained my calf, and as I stood looking at the vast painting, it throbbed and pulsed with pain. See how fragile we are?

The weather is stormy and I sit in the premier lounge at Marco Polo airport watching lightning miss planes by inches. How much alcohol should I drink? If Jesus were here . . . but of course Jesus would not be in the premier lounge at Marco Polo airport. For the next few hours I try to play the "What would Jesus do?" game. But would Jesus really go on a getaway to Venice? Would Jesus cry because he had to go on a bus in a thunderstorm for five minutes? Would Jesus, when faced with a barrier attendant at St. Pancras who asks to see his railcard, first argue that since other people don't have to show their railcards when going through the normal barriers, it does not make any sense to single out only the people with the most luggage who need to go through the wider barriers, and then eventually tell her to fuck off? If Jesus played tennis he would win all the time. But I bet Jesus would not play tennis. Jesus would have better things to do.

But of course one of the reasons—or are these becoming excuses?—for playing tennis in the first place is spiritual. Forget winning and losing. Sport is about endurance, patience, doing your best. It's about being a good competitor. Breathing. Achieving flow. Getting in the zone. It's about using the body to leave the body behind. Transcending the self. But I am not transcending the self. I am so bogged down in my own ego that I think I might be on the verge of going under. I have started equating winning with being loved and accepted. I take everything personally, even the good stuff. When Dan texts me to say he can play with me on the Saturday after I get back, I'm thrilled. I can't wait to get on the court. The beautiful green acrylic and the echoes and the zip and thud of the ball. But I'm also really pleased he has remembered and is not cross about the Josh thing.

I love tennis with Dan when we listen to music and just hit. I also like playing points with him. But anything that looks like a drill makes me feel like a baby, especially as he's not even my coach anymore—not that he knows this, of course. I am becoming bad at taking instruction from him. And Dan really overdoes it in our first session back. I tell him I want to learn a two-handed backhand, partly to distract him, and partly to cover up the fact that I have already done the basics with Josh. I really just want to whack the ball back and forth, but instead we have long conversations about grips and footwork. But I guess it's fine, and I feel guilty about the whole Josh thing anyway, and my backhand is coming on. Dan is not, I don't think, suspicious. I have a session booked with Josh for Monday morning at 9:00 a.m. Josh and I both know Dan isn't even out of bed then, so he doesn't need to be told just yet.

At the end of the session we're picking up balls from the back of the court. We're kind of chatting about the Canterbury Open— officially called the Advantage RedCourt East Kent Junior and Adult Championships. It's a Grade 4 that I'm definitely going to enter. It's essentially the next big local tournament after the Spring Open. And the next one after that will be the Walmer Open in August, which doesn't carry LTA ranking points but everyone plays in anyway.

"I think I'm going to join the club at Canterbury as well," I say. "What do you think?"

Dan picks up a ball and uses his racquet to slam-crash it into the black curtain at the back of the court.

"You going to play for Polo?" he asks. Canterbury Tennis Club is based at Polo Farm.

"I don't know. I don't think so."

Dan bends down to pick up a particularly battered green ball. "We could join together," he says. "Have some hits on clay. That would be good."

"OK . . ."

"Of course, it wouldn't be right if any money changed hands. It would be just, you know, just as friends."

He doesn't meet my eye when he stands up. We both know this is a big deal. And then he does look at me. Flashes me a little shy smile.

"So?"

"Um, oh, yes! Of course. That would be amazing!"

Wow. Fuck. OK. Someone as good as Dan wants to play with me for fun, for free, as a friend. I am childishly thrilled. Of course this is what I've been hoping for ages, but I never knew how, or even if, it might happen. Even though I don't seem to be able to win any actual matches, I do seem to be improving.

•

Of course, I am the organized one, the one with money and resources and willingness to fill in forms in the name of tennis. So by the next afternoon, I have rung the membership secretary of Canterbury Tennis Club and I'm going down for a practice hit (and I think to be vetted) the following day. The Membership Secretary, Judith, is the same as last time I played here, but I doubt she'll remember me. In those days I was so rubbish I might as well have not even existed. Now I have a ranking and a rating and everything.

The practice hit goes well, I think. Judith puts me on with her and two other mild-looking ladies who look startled when I grunt and try to poach at the net and hit crosscourt winners. After I hit a few nice topspin shots down the tramlines, I am put on to play with a tall, freckled builder named Del. He's probably in his late fifties or early sixties, but has the vibe of someone who has been a member of this club for at least a hundred years. We play two other men, recreational players of about my age with paunches and the haunted looks of those who at this moment should really be working, shopping, looking after a toddler, pouring Chardonnay for a harassed wife.

For some reason I don't know, we're playing the best of eight games, but the other groups' games go on and so therefore we do too.

In the end we beat them 8–0.

Afterward, Del wants to know where I've come from. I tell him I play in the leagues for the leisure center and he seems impressed.

"You should play for us," he says. "You should play for the ladies' First Team."

Before I leave, I fill in the form for membership and leave it with Judith. She says I can come in the next day to pick up my key fob and get my password for the computer booking system. I ask for a second form.

"My mixed doubles partner wants to join as well," I say proudly. "Maybe you know Dan Brewer? He's a coach at the leisure center."

Judith shakes her head, but gives me another form anyway.

Dan isn't in a hurry to fill it out, though. It sits on his desk for days, seemingly lost in a pile of sandwich containers and kids' report forms. As a member of Canterbury LTC, I can have a guest—I think a maximum of three times a season—as long as I put £5 in the tub in the clubhouse. So the first time we play, Dan is there as my guest.

Not that you'd think so, though. Dan seems to know everyone. He stops and chats with a guy named Chuck, and then someone named Steve. Simon, the head coach at Canterbury, is hitting balls to a tiny wiry dark-haired girl of about eleven, and when they stop for a break, he comes over and says hello to Dan, who doesn't introduce me. In fact, both of them ignore me. Dan seems mildly stressed and unlike himself.

Never mind. Eventually we go onto our court.

"Wow. It's, like, grainy," Dan says of the artificial clay.

"You have played on it before, right?"

"Nope," he says. "Do you really have to sweep it?"

"Yep. With real brooms. So you know Simon, then?" I say, noticing that Dan keeps glancing over at him.

"Yeah, I'm like . . ."

"What?"

Dan lowers his voice. "Don't say anything, but I'm really scared of him. I literally can't play badly while he's watching."

"He's not watching. He's coaching that girl."

"Do you know who that is?"

"No. Who?"

"Tiegan Aitken. He coaches her all the time. For free. She's going to be like number one in the country. She's number one in county juniors at the moment."

I feel unspeakably jealous all of sudden.

My dream. *My* dream. It's not that it was even unattainable: people are living it all around me. It's just that I never got to live it. Well, all that can still change, right?

When we start playing, it's terrible. Dan clearly doesn't want to be shown up playing with a recreational lady, so he slams the ball wildly all over the court while making unamusing banter and generally showing off. Two courts away from us, Simon shows no signs of noticing. I know this, because of course I'm trying to show off too. What if Simon did notice me, like, properly? He's already turned me down for coaching, yes, but that was before he knew who I was. I imagine playing one of my perfect backhands down the line, or the crosscourt forehand winner that Dan always complains about, and Simon noticing and then talking to me afterward and offering to train me for international seniors' competitions or whatever would interest him most. I get so lost in my fantasy that I don't look around for ages and when I do, he and Tiegan have gone.

After that, Dan settles down too and we have quite a nice hit, although he thrashes me in the first game we play for points.

I've noticed that when we cross at the net after the first game of a set, when it's customary to just change ends without sitting down, Dan never goes first. I assumed it was politeness, but today I sense something more.

"You go," I say, stepping aside and gesturing.

"No, you."

"Why won't you go first?"

"It's just a thing I've got," he says. "If I cross the net first, something bad'll happen."

"What, you'll lose?"

"No. Something worse."

In the next drinks break, I tell Dan about Luke Green, the coach here who I only hit with, of course, fucking up so many of his serves and overheads. I say that Luke hits the ball in the net way more often than Dan does.

"Tosser," says Dan, jealously.

"*Dan*," I chide.

"And you're sure he doesn't actually coach you? It's just hitting?"

"Of course. I told you."

This is very sweet in its own way, but does not make me inclined to bring up Josh, which I really have to do soon, before we are found out.

Dan takes the first set 6–1, which is kind of depressing. But I remind myself that Sharapova came back from that against Halep in Madrid last week. Nadal will do the same thing against Andy Murray later today, although obviously I don't know that yet. I focus on my game plan—hit deep to his backhand at all times—and actually get ahead in the next set, 4–3. Dan takes the next two games and although I get a point away from making it 5–5 he takes the set 6–4. I'm happy with that.

Dan is off to see Steve Davis performing in Ashford and is running late, so I agree to take his completed membership form down to the office. It's a miracle that he's remembered to do it at all. Obviously on the way I read it. I want to see what he's written in the part where you have to describe your standard of play. I expect him to have put something like AWESOME TENNIS COACH in capital letters, or at least to have said something about being head coach at both the Indoor Tennis Centre and Folkestone. But instead it's rather modest: "9.2, reasonable doubles player, currently playing in Kent and East Kent leagues." But then he is modest, unlike me.

•

I've suffered from anxiety for most of my life. It got a lot worse after the abortion, but I'd be lying if I tried to blame it all on that. I can't exactly blame my family complications either. When Mum and Gordian sat down with me when I was twelve and told me Gordian was my father, I was dazed and kind of pleased. Finally, something interesting had happened to me! I was probably most affected by Mum's breakup with Steve when I was nine. When we first moved to Chelmsford I would lie in bed and imagine fires and floods and other natural disasters. I made the family do fire drills and felt thankful that we didn't have those double-glazed windows that people couldn't escape from. I would usually go to sleep terrified that something bad was going to happen overnight and I would never wake up. But even before that I'd been quite a timid child, afraid of the dark, ghosts, being on my own.

My anxiety has come and gone over the years. I've learned that I am worse if I have too much caffeine, alcohol, and sugar, and also, of course, when I am stressed. After we moved to our current seaside town in 2010, I was worried it was a mistake. It was just a bit too far from the university—a forty-five-minute drive that I would do too early with wet hair to try to beat the traffic and get a parking space. I was full-time then, running Creative Writing at Kent. This sounds grander than it was. Creative Writing occupies its own unique little space in the university—semi-independent but part of the School of English. It was like the professional equivalent of being a teenager who's been given a small allowance. Every time a big decision needed to be made, someone else had to do it—often someone who wasn't even as senior as me, but occupied a big admin role in the wider School of English.

Soon I developed a psychological problem with one part of the road into work: a long straight narrow section on which people drove a bit too fast. Eventually, I would shake and cry whenever I had to drive down it—or worse, my vision would blur and I'd be convinced I would pass out. What if I completely lost it and drove onto the wrong side of the road? What if I did it when a big lorry or bus was coming? What if I did it on purpose, in a terrible moment of madness? What was wrong with me? It was then that I signed up for the sessions with the transpersonal therapist who got me thinking about *A Course in Miracles* and being loved. It helped to unleash Scary Scarlett, but it genuinely enhanced my spirituality too. My thing with the road faded in the end and I felt a bit better. Reducing my hours and not being Director of Creative Writing helped even more, and led me to wonder whether giving up the university altogether would be better for my mental health.

Now, I'm not sure what tennis is doing to it.

The following Sunday is our first Aegon away match in Maidstone. We're playing a team called LA Fitness Ladies. I imagine big boobs and high-cut rainbow-colored leotards. I plan a long circuitous route that will take about two hours but at least doesn't involve motorways. Like my mother, I never drive on motorways. I completely freak out if I find myself on one: like the scene in *Clueless*, but not funny. My neck goes numb, then my arms, then my vision starts to blur.

Somehow, I don't feel right the whole way to Maidstone. When I drive across a bridge over the M2 (the very motorway I'm specifically not driving on), I get a sudden vertiginous urge to throw myself off it. I think that if I had to stop here and contemplate the void below, I'd find it so painful I'd have to throw myself in. It's basically vertigo, but on a motorway bridge. What the fuck? Until recently, all my anxieties have been about things outside myself. A fire, an earthquake, a plane crash. I used to insist on driving everywhere myself because I didn't trust other drivers of any sort. But what happens if you can't trust yourself? What if the problem is inside you, not outside? But the feeling passes quickly and I don't think about it again for a while.

It takes ages to get to Maidstone the way I'm going, but it is a beautiful hot day, and I'm listening to cheap pop music on Heart FM, and once the anxiety about the motorway bridge passes, I feel pretty good. I love playing tennis in the heat: it's one of my strengths. While visiting teams visibly wilt and complain that they feel faint in the ITC, I seem to be a pure machine running only on Evian water. I sweat like Nadal, like some kind of permanent spurting fountain, and then I simply replace all my fluids. It's fine; pleasurable even. Later, when everything goes wrong, one of my theories about what's wrong with me will be dehydration, and then I'll realize that I should put a pinch of salt in my water, or a fizzy pink electrolyte tablet. But now? I do none of that.

LA Fitness is quite hard to find, and Siri isn't much help. I drive around the one-way system a couple of times before realizing I have to go under an old Victorian railway bridge and into an industrial estate and then down a narrow concrete lane. It's all cheerful, light and plastic inside, like a kind of dry swimming pool. There's a brightly lit bar and some glossy suburban mothers and a couple of sulky teenage girls.

Fiona is waiting for me. She's with Jane, the captain of LA Fitness Ladies.

"Well, it's just us," Fiona says.

"What do you mean?"

She shrugs. "Margaret literally couldn't find anyone else to play. She didn't even tell me. She phoned Jane."

Jane nods. "That's right."

"But why didn't we cancel?" I say.

"It's not fair to cancel altogether," says Jane. "I mean, the girls want a game. And we've made a lot of afternoon tea."

For God's sake. I'm fuming. Maidstone is not exactly around the fucking corner. With only two players we can't win or even draw.

We should have just canceled and given LA Fitness the points. Of course, I never ended up captaining this Aegon team: Margaret decided to captain herself, which is fair enough. And somehow Becky ended up playing for us as well—at least, she's apparently down for this game but can't play. And Margaret has apparently been roped into working at the ITC and no one else was available, not even Kofo or Karen or Hayley.

"Margaret thought we'd want the games too," says Fiona. "I mean, I bloody don't. It's my husband's birthday today."

"Yeah, and I've got to go to a dinner party in Faversham later. I could have done without this."

Jane puts the two teenage girls, Lucy and Gabby, on against Fiona and me. We have to play singles first, then the doubles. My opponent Gabby is fifteen years old and a 5.1. This isn't what I came here for. Although I suppose as an 8.2 I would have probably had to play her anyway, because I'm the highest rated in my team. But what's a 5.1 doing in League 2 of Kent Aegon Team Tennis? Maybe League 1 is full of 2.1s and 1.2s. Unlikely, though, given that players of that standard would be playing national tournaments. Given the circumstances, it would be fairer and more fun for me and Fiona to play the older women. LA Fitness Ladies has won anyway. But no.

Gabby has beautiful pale blue eyes, high cheekbones, and shoulders made entirely of right angles. Oh, well. I've been here before. I don't even need to give myself permission to lose, as it seems inevitable. I begin tight and embarrassed and still a bit annoyed because it would have been so much more fun to play the older women on the team. This is Vanessa Brill all over again. Gabby's mother is watching, but there are other people too. A brother? Her father? They clap her good shots and call her Gabs. Everyone loves her. No one loves me. I have become an extra in Gabs's life. Except she is having trouble returning my first serve, and not because it's rubbish, either. If I hit to her forehand she kills it, but her backhand is not so strong. I keep to my game plan and play to her backhand as often as possible. In the end it's 6–1, 6–1. But I am pleased that the two games I get are my service games and I win them properly. I am quite happy with my serve. I managed to return her serve well. I got good depth on a lot of my shots. And I am really loving playing in the heat, as I knew I would. But otherwise this is fucking depressing and so, so pointless.

Before we begin the doubles, the parents open a bottle of Chardonnay. They stand there in the shade, glasses of wine in hand, as the girls thrash us 6–0, 6–2. There is no shade on these courts, not even a tiny bit to stand in when we change ends. It doesn't take long, but by the time we've finished, the parents are on to a second bottle of wine. After the match is over, we go into the bar and they, and the non-playing members of the team, order more wine, rosé this time. Afternoon tea is laid out on one of the low round tables in the bar area. It's 100 percent wheat: cakes, sandwiches, pretzels.

"Oh God, I'm really sorry. I should have said I was gluten-free," I say.

Jane glowers at me. "Those cakes are homemade," she says.

"Come on," says Fiona. "We'll have to try and eat some of it."

So I sit there eating Victoria sponge cake while Gabby's and Lucy's parents congratulate them and ask them about their training and their GCSEs and no one says anything to me at all.

•

I think Rod's a bit pissed off with me. Why wouldn't he be? After all, I am now obsessed with tennis to the exclusion of all else. We did manage a holiday, but I spent the whole thing reading tennis books, missing tennis, and thinking about going back to tennis. Which is why I've agreed to this dinner party I don't want to go to, with his friends in Faversham. The deal is that we don't stay long and he drives. There will be nice people there: Abdulrazak Gurnah and Denise Narian are good friends, and I always love seeing them. Then there's Lyn Innes and Martin Schofield. I'm opposite Martin. Everyone's into my tennis adventure, and I'm happy to talk about it. One great thing about tennis is it means I'm not socially awkward anymore. I always, always have conversation.

This evening, though, I'm fucking knackered. Yes, I do have my usual chilled post-exercise buzz, but it increasingly now flattens too quickly into exhaustion, into a state where I can only just keep going without knowing exactly what fuel I'm running on. But wait, I do know: it's alcohol. After a couple of glasses of white wine, I feel a bit more sparkly, but when I go into the downstairs loo I'm sure everyone can hear me yelp as I try to sit on it to pee. It's my knees. They are so tight and achy. And my quads. And my hamstrings. And my calves. My arm feels a lot better, though.

When I get back, Martin's saying something about Laurence Goldstein, a colleague from another department in the university. I instinctively cue up my favorite Laurence story, although there are lots. My second favorite is from when I was on an appointments panel with Laurence for a lectureship in philosophy and we'd just finished reading the harrowing story of one applicant: a single mother who'd been disabled after a car accident and then found she had cancer.

"Well, she's going to be a right whinger," said Laurence into the awkward silence, with his perfect comic timing. It was exactly what you can't say, what you're not supposed to say, but what everyone's thinking. And because Laurence was so kind and gentle, he could get away with saying things like that—just throwing a bit of honesty out there and seeing what came back.

But my favorite Laurence story is from just after the university decided to shut down the Center for Divination, a part of the Religious Studies department.

"They should have seen it coming," said Laurence, with a cheeky grin.

Laurence joined the university the year after me, in 2005. He'd had a world-renowned academic post in Hong Kong just before that and had joined Kent as a professor. Being a novelist and, as I was at that time, a cricketer means you make all sorts of unusual connections around the university. I knew people from the Business School, Computing, Anthropology. One of my closest cricketing friends, Mudassar Iqbal, was working on a computer program that could predict the effects of certain viruses and hormones in the body. I think I first met Laurence because I was trying to get him to play on the staff cricket team. Or maybe it was because he, as a paradox-solving polymath, also roamed the university meeting new and different people and wanted to talk to me about paradoxes. He set up a Centre for Paradox and for a while four of us would meet and talk about how paradox was important in our particular disciplines. I planned to talk about paradox in *Hamlet* but never quite got around to it. In those days I was younger and more enthusiastic about the university. I wanted to know people, do things, be someone.

I haven't seen Laurence for months, but he recently sent me a book through interoffice post about sport that I haven't got around to reading yet. Last time I saw him he talked about how he wished he could swap the years he spent training as an elite cyclist for extra time to think about philosophy and Wittgenstein. I argued at the time that sport *is* pure philosophy: it means actually living, properly striving and struggling. I probably declared that it is Nietzschean; Dionysian.

"Yes," Martin is saying, across the dinner table. "It's an inoperable brain tumor."

"What?" I say. "Laurence? Not really?"

"Oh yes," says Martin in his smooth, don't-care, dinner-party voice. "He's expected to die at any moment."

On the way home I try to cry, but I'm too shocked. When I do cry it's not for Laurence exactly—it hasn't completely sunk in, and I'm not even sure I believe it's that bad—it's for me, and for what I've lost. I used to be a real part of the university. I knew people. I played for the staff cricket team. I'm not exactly sure what happened, but I had no idea I'd disconnected to quite this extent, that a dear professional friend could be this ill and me not know about it at all.

The next day an email goes around saying that Laurence has died.

•

In my office I sit there, drained and hungover, thinking about Laurence. I'm also trying to write an email to Dan confessing that Josh is now my coach. I can't do it. Should I cancel my next session with Josh? Then again, it's not as if Dan will stop playing with Hayley Palmer because I'm jealous of her. And what about that time he laughed and joked with her at the Monday session and more or less ignored me? But I know that it's not the same. Anyway, Dan and I are playing together in the Canterbury tournament. It's all settled. We're going to enter the mixed doubles part of the tournament together! But can friends claim total exclusivity? Isn't it a bit unreasonable that

Dan should want me to hit with him and only him? Although, again, I know this isn't the case. Dan doesn't care who I play with as long as it isn't other coaches. And of course, the other thing is that I am lying to Dan. I am telling him it will only be a hit with Josh, when in fact I want Josh to secretly teach me things. Is it noble to be going this far to spare Dan's feelings or am I simply trying to make myself feel better? I feel fourteen years old again, in a bad way.

After work I go to Polo Farm for a hit with Luke. He's in a bit of a weird mood today and talking about how he wants to stop doing cardio and start doing more CrossFit and weightlifting: how he needs to put on muscle. He's quite a skinny guy, but athletic-looking and attractive. I've been thinking that part of my yoga-teacher role with men might be to coach them on their fitness goals a bit, so I'm interested in what Luke's trying to do. I also try to reassure him.

"I mean, you already look like something from a feature in *Men's Health*," I say kindly. Who wouldn't want that, right?

"Yeah." He looks a bit tortured. "Ideally I want to look like someone on the cover. Like, in fact actually *be* the guy on the cover." Right.

We hit outside on clay and then play some points. Surprisingly, I beat him 4–3. It's a miracle, especially as the usual conversation in my head starts when I am 3–1 up. I imagine telling Rod, and Dan, and now Josh as well, that I beat a twenty-four-year-old male coach at Polo Farm. Of course, the more I do this, the more I lose points and games, but Luke only gets it to 3–4 before our time is up. Can I only beat people who are falling apart in some way? Luke is clearly struggling with something. He serves double faults galore and hits the ball wide and I get many, many points for free.

"Oh well," he says afterward. "At least I'm trying to play my game."

"Yeah," I say. "Anyway, it's not important who wins."

"I'm just trying to practice for the tournament, really," he says.

"Yeah, me too."

"I'm playing a 9.2 in the first round," Luke says. "So I should beat him easy."

"Always watch out for 9.2s," I say.

"It'll be all right as long as he's not a pusher," says Luke. "Or a dibbly-dobbler."

"Yeah. Fuck. I hate that."

"It's impossible to play against them."

"Yeah, but I guess really good players don't have any problem with them." It sounds worse than I mean it to, but it's true. If being a dibbly-dobbler really made you unbeatable, then it's the kind of tennis Andy Murray would play. Evolution would mean that people would focus on developing that style, if it was really the most unbeatable.

"True," says Luke. "The key is not being dragged down to their level."

•

It's finally Monday, May 26, the first day of the Canterbury tournament. I've entered everything: the women's singles, which has seven entries; the mixed doubles, which has three entries; and, with Siobhan Clarke, the ladies' doubles, which has six entries. I'm not on until tomorrow, but Siobhan is playing this evening. Also, the other two mixed doubles pairs are going head-to-head and I decide it will be fun to watch them. I'm so excited by this idea of a real tournament that will take place over a whole week. Rod's interested too. He's going to come and we'll make an evening of it somehow.

When Rod and I arrive, Luke Green is just about to play a guy named Lloyd Daniels. I know he's from Sandwich because just before they begin he shouts, "Come on the Sandwich!" half to himself and half to what must be his doubles partner, who is sitting watching him. Lloyd's fiftyish; the partner, Stuart, is a bit younger. The sky is a whitish gray and a steady mizzle is falling on all the players. Lloyd must be the 9.2 that Luke was talking about. He's hilarious. He keeps up a constant dialogue with himself and the few spectators. *What a talent!* he declares as he serves a double fault. *You goof!* he says when he hits the ball in the net. He calls himself a gimp, an idiot, a buffoon. Also, he keeps going on about his lunch, experiencing it all over again. He does not move his feet but has a surprisingly robust forehand and quite a penetrating one-handed backhand. Luke has another psychological collapse and loses 6–3, 6–4, after which he storms off.

The next match I'm interested in is Siobhan Clarke versus Sue Depledge. *Forgive me,* I think as it gets going, *but please say I don't play like that!* It's pure dibbly-dobbly tennis, the ball moving slowly in the half-light, moonball after moonball after moonball. On the next court over I can see Teele Annus, the twenty-three-year-old top seed for the women's singles and one half of the mixed team Dan and I will face on Thursday, warming up for her first mixed match. This is more like it. Proper shots. She moves her feet. Her left arm does not dangle uselessly by her side when she plays her nice topspin forehand. She's young, blonde, and Nordic looking. Quite hot. A proper player. She's a 6.1, but looks better than that.

Sue Depledge eventually beats Siobhan after a long, boring battle. Sue wins the first set pretty easily, 6–2, like a cancer taking hold. But Siobhan is good at fighting back and takes the second set 7–5, like a big dose of radiotherapy. The championship tiebreak in lieu of a third set is like a long bout of chemo that goes to 10–7. But poor Siobhan loses her fight. She looks like she'd rather be dead. When she comes off court she's all smiles until Sue goes to get in her estate car to drive home.

"God," says Siobhan. "I hate it when people take the pace off the ball."

"Yeah," I agree. "So hard to play against dibbly-dobblers."

Sue is a middle-aged woman with a focused, intense look about her. Is it just her lack of pace that means she wins? When I get home I look her up on the LTA website and discover that she was born in 1967 and is a 7.2. Astonishingly, she is the number 10 player over forty in the whole country! How the actual fuck is that possible? I'm sure she's an extremely lovely person, but cutting-edge power tennis she is not. Maybe it was just the rain, or where I was sitting, or some weird combo effect with Siobhan, but actually, she looked pretty awful.

Instead of thinking that her stats mean that these rankings mean nothing and are not worth achieving, I immediately start plotting my own route to the top. I mean, this is totally doable, right? If she's number 10, then I could easily get to number 5, right? I wonder how long it would take me. And then I could push on into the top three. Could I be the top player in my age group in the country? The world? OK, probably not the world, but I could be disciplined and focused and I'd never, ever have to prove myself again. I'd always have tales of my glory for dinner parties and book events. I'd never have to wait for a book review to tell me I'm worthwhile: I'd have numbers to do it for me. Real, concrete, beautiful numbers. And that sweet, sweet emotional combination of victory and happy tiredness all the time.

Tuesday afternoon, and it's raining steadily. As Rod and I set off, we wonder whether there'll be any tennis at all, or whether the tournament may have moved inside. But when we get to Polo Farm, the clay courts are all steamed up with bodies and heavy, fluffy tennis balls. Lina and Carol from Canterbury come off after beating Sara and Gaye from Sandwich. Siobhan has come to watch me, which is nice of her. She's wearing a fluffy pink sweater with a heart on it and carrying a copy of *Closer* magazine. I'm to play Sarah Philips, 9.2, a solid Canterbury club player. I'm told she's not expected to win anything but has just entered because she loves the club, and there are never enough women for the Open Women's Singles.

We're given a tube of balls and sent to Court 1. The floodlights are on and it's still drizzling at 6:30, when we begin. Sarah's less nervous than me and takes the first two games but then I come back, and after a lot of wet, cold rallies we're playing a tiebreak for the first set. I save a set point against me by serving an ace down the T into the ad court, which feels pretty cool. I get myself to 6–5 but can't close it out. What's wrong with me that I can't do this? Why can't I just keep serving aces? I am developing a thing about tiebreaks. Sarah takes it and—fuck, fuck, fuck—we're into the second set. And I'm a set down. Crap. Crapola. Crapadoodledoo.

In the break, Rod looks at me and gestures that I should hit out more. No shit, Sherlock.

We go back on. I decide that I've lost now and I don't care and then I relax and as usual that's when my best tennis comes out. I take the first three games easily. I've been serving well throughout, but now Sarah really can't return my serve to the deuce side. And if she moves slightly wide to receive it, I blast it down the T. She comes back for two games but somehow I manage to close out the set and take it 6–2. This is more like it. Why couldn't I have done that in the first set? Anyway, I'm clearly the stronger player. This is amazing. All I have to do is take my momentum into the tiebreak and win.

But alas, in my last service game of the second set both my calves began to cramp and are getting steadily worse. In the break I glug water and eat some crisps and ask for a bit of extra time, but it's getting really dark now—we've been at it for almost two hours. This is ridiculous. Why a fucking injury, now? I tell myself I can't possibly win, especially as it turns out I'm cramping so much I can't serve or run at all. But of course if I do win I'll be into the next round—the actual semifinals—with some ranking points, playing Teele Annus. And I *am* the stronger player, but I can't think that. I can't think I'm going to win, or I will lose.

While I wrestle with myself, someone finds some tokens and puts on the floodlights. In the milky orange light a confused bird starts to sing, out of place, out of time. *Like me*, I think.

I lose the tiebreak 8–10. On the last couple of points I am in agony. At one point I fall to the ground clutching my leg, not for drama but for real. I literally cannot move. When we shake hands at the net, Sarah apologizes, because she can see how injured I am. *Give me the victory then*, I think in my head. *You know I deserve it.* But of course that isn't how this works. On the way home I feel so sad and deflated. I won more real games—twelve, to Sarah's eight— but managed to lose two tiebreaks and with them the match. Was it because of my cramp? Would I have fucked it up anyway? At some point in the match I realized that if I lost I'd have to play Siobhan Clarke again, which I really don't want to do. But now I am.

Still, when I get home around 10:00 p.m., wet and cold, I quite enjoy the process of unpacking my bag and throwing the things I'll need for tomorrow into the washing machine and starting the whole thing again. I lost today but I'll win tomorrow, right? I'll make a game plan and it'll be fine. I have my forehand. My serve. My muscles. My fitness. My calves will be OK. I'm still in a tournament!

Before bed I check out everyone else's scores. Lloyd the buffoon lost 6–3, 6–1 to the top seed, Graham Hunt. Their match had been taking place on the court next to mine and at one point I'd wondered from his jolly commentary if he was actually winning. Meanwhile, Meredith Willicombe-Lang, the strong-looking Black girl I last saw beating Charanya Ravi in the first round at Leicester, got a walkover because the second seed, Allessia Cuomo, didn't show up.

Wednesday. I have not seen the sky for days. Rod and I are going to Laurence's funeral before Rod drops me off at Polo Farm and goes back for the wake. I've got to play doubles with Siobhan. I can't let her down.

Rod told me once about a theory that at each funeral you attend you are actually reacting to the one before. Perhaps this explains why I completely fall apart as soon as I walk in to Laurence's. I didn't even cry at Steve's funeral. Why? Was it because I was so busy worrying about Sam and helping him to run the whole thing? Afterward, we had to clear out Steve's squalid house in Gloucester where everything was filthy and broken, syringes strewn all over the floor. Amidst the horror was a battered copy of *The End of Mr. Y*, and a hardback of my follow-up, *Our Tragic Universe*. I didn't know how to process this. I still don't. It turned out that Steve had been so proud of me that he'd always kept up the fiction that I was his daughter.

And then sixteen days later Dreamer died and I never got over it.

At Laurence's funeral, "Penny Lane" by the Beatles is playing. The place is packed. I'm given a funeral program with a picture of Laurence on the front. I simply can't believe this man is dead. I can't believe that I have got so out of touch with the university that I didn't even know he was dying until the day before it happened. The last time I saw him I was in a hurry and didn't even really say hello. I never thanked him for the book he sent me. I was a bad friend.

I can't stop crying. It's uncontrollable. I'm crying for Dreamer, for Steve, for my whole past, and my present, and my weight that won't move and my stupid cramping calves and everything that went wrong in my childhood and every tennis match I've ever lost.

As the service goes on, I calm down a little and start wondering if I am a good mourner, if I am winning at mourning. Has anyone noticed how much I am crying? If so, will they know how genuine it is? Should I cry more to make sure? No, but that's stupid, because that isn't genuine anymore. I wonder if anyone will notice that Scarlett Thomas, the famous novelist, is here crying at the funeral of a man most people wouldn't realize she knew quite well and deeply understood, a man who always made her laugh, whose irreverence was a beautiful light shining through the university. I try to stop thinking these thoughts, but I somehow can't. Everything I do is a competition. Everything I do is a performance. Everything I do has a commentary.

And then I'm back at Polo Farm, still clutching a shredded tissue and with all my eye makeup gone, stepping out in the gloom to play doubles with Siobhan against Sarah Philips and Elaine Povey. I can't do this. I am too sad. My body feels heavy. I've had no time to warm up. I haven't eaten enough. I haven't had any ibuprofen. My hand hurts. I can hardly hit a tennis ball and I don't even care. We lose the first set quickly, 1–6. That's OK. I told Siobhan we were going to get annihilated. I mean, this is my home turf, and I sort of know these players. I've heard they are good. And Siobhan and I have never played together.

But somehow, as the set has gone on the games have got longer and my ibuprofen has kicked in and Siobhan is serving really well and it gradually dawns on me that she can play doubles. In fact, she's rather good. We take the first game in the second set, then the next one. I'm playing on the ad side, which I like. Usually the stronger doubles player goes on the ad side, because there are more backhands, but because Hannah Martin is left-handed I always play on the deuce side with her, and also, of course, with Dan. Anyway, this is a chance to practice my inside-out forehand, which is very cool. It's when you are on the ad side of the court trading crosscourt backhands but your opponent sends a slower, weaker, less-angled one that you are able to step around, as if you're stepping out of the way of someone about to walk into you on a busy street, and hit as a forehand instead. You still hit this crosscourt to their backhand, but with the strength and speed of a forehand. It's more or less guaranteed to be a winner, or set one up.

I use Josh's new western grip—shake hands with the racquet as every kid knows how to do, but then keep turning my wrist to the right until it feels odd—and keep my elbow up. It doesn't matter, as we're going to lose this match anyway. I start attacking Elaine's serve, which freaks her out. I play aggressive forehands low to her backhand when she is at the net. She fluffs them all, then gets frustrated with herself, which means I do it more. I smash some balls away at the net. We're on fire—we take the set 6–4. All-out aggression is actually amazing.

Time for another championship tiebreak. Rod arrives, looking fragile and beautiful in his old anorak. If I lost him, it would be—I would be—it has started to rain again. My thoughts start to drizzle steadily along with it. We are 7–3 up in the tiebreak when I realize that if we win this, we're in the final. And I thought we were going to be wiped out so easily. Of course, this is exactly when we stop winning points. I double-fault and then spin a couple of easy back-hands into the net. Siobhan, perhaps picking up my bad vibes, or maybe with nerves of her own, fluffs a couple of volleys. Somewhere in all this we get another point, but they get their momentum back and win 10–8. I really, really hate championship tiebreaks. And I don't understand why the most innocent thought of winning makes me lose.

Still, I'm relaxed going straight into my ladies' singles match with Siobhan in the first round of the consolation draw. We're both feeling pleased with our very first doubles performance. I'm loving the powerful feeling my forehand is giving me. My game plan with Siobhan was to go all-out aggressive against what I thought might be steady, dibbly-dobbly play. But in fact *she* is aggressive and therefore making mistakes, so I play with a bit more "controlled" aggression. Am I the one dibbly-dobbling? No. Well, I'm trying not to go that far. I hit hard and deep to her backhand and manage to win a few good points with my down-the-line forehand. A few times I follow a short ball into the net but she passes or lobs me. I remind myself that I should go into the net off one of my own approach shots, not hers. I realize I'm winning more points from the baseline, so I camp out there.

My calves are still not recovered and feel 60 percent at most, and as a result I don't really have my first serve. It's raining harder and there are little insects everywhere, swooping and dipping in the so-dium lights. My Adidas tights are annoying me; I wish I'd worn my Falke ones. I somehow take the first set 6–3. It should have been 6–2, but I couldn't close out on my serve and had to break hers instead. But it's fine, right? I'm winning so easily, after all. To make her feel better on the changeover, I say I prefer playing her to Sarah because she hits it harder and more aggressively. Why the fuck did I say that? I worry that she'll do her old trick of taking the pace off the ball now, but surely it doesn't matter because I am on fire.

She wins the next set 6–0. I'm not even sure how she does it. Rod says that I was the one who stopped playing so aggressively. That's not how it felt. Siobhan certainly played a whole lot better, but how? Afterward I don't even know whether she took the pace off the ball or not. It feels like some kind of voodoo or a hex. Rod keeps saying that to him it seemed that she was playing more strongly and I was the one who backed off. Why did I stop hitting the ball hard? My legs felt bad, I know that. But not so bad I couldn't play. Did my thoughts do it again? I'd told myself to win the first set if I wanted to avoid a championship tiebreak and then I'd done it. It simply didn't occur to me that I could win a first set and then lose the second. I'd been thinking instead how obvious it is now that I am better than Siobhan, that all my hard work and coaching has paid off, and that the Spring Open was just an anomaly, or a painful but necessary step on the road leading here, to a 6–3, 6–2 (maybe) victory and another match against maybe Sue or Meredith and some ranking points.

This is ridiculous. Any thoughts of winning at all and I lose. What is so wrong with me that I seem to have to reach an egoless higher state of calm and detachment before I can win anything? Other people can win without having to achieve enlightenment first. Why can't I? Presumably Sarah wanted to win, thought about winning? Siobhan clearly *really* wanted to win. I doubt they spend too much time meditating and reading *The Inner Game of Tennis*. Or maybe they do, and the reason I lose is because I underestimate everybody. Why can't I just win once? *Please?* Is it that I want it too much, or not enough? Do I feel guilty about winning? Not worthy of it? Or am I just not good enough? If I had a few more winning shots? Am I just unlucky? Cramp in one match. Playing after a funeral. Drinking too much. Not drinking enough. Playing on clay. Playing on carpet. Playing on macadam. Did I have enough protein before this match? No, I didn't have any. I've recently given up dairy products. Should I have had some?

When I get home, I check the scores from the other matches. Luke lost in the consolation draw against a 10.2 opponent, 6–0, 6–1. And he lost his doubles too. Why is seeing someone do worse than you so comforting? Is it a bad thing? Maybe not. I respect Luke, and I know he's a good player. If he can fuck up this bad then anyone can. It's just one of those things. But I still feel like a complete loser. How can I not win even one match? How is it possible that with all my training and dedication I am probably going to come *last* in a local Grade 4?

Oh well. There's always the mixed doubles.

The mixed doubles is a round robin and both our matches are on Thursday. The first one, against Teele Annus and Matt Brears, is at 4:00 p.m. At last, the sun has come out. I'm looking forward to winning a match at last. Not the first one obviously, but the second one, against Sara Fairclough and Joseph Sevier from Sandwich. We're playing that today as well, right after the first match.

At ten to four Dan has still not arrived and I'm starting to get worried. The nice thing about doubles is you have a partner to warm up with and talk to and have a hit with before you go on—if you're not rushing from a funeral, that is. Dan isn't rushing from a funeral. Where is he? A few minutes later I get a text saying he's running late from his Level 4 training day. Of course—that's what he's been doing. At ten past four he rolls in like a wounded hero, all droopy and pathetic, talking about having gotten up at 5:00 a.m. to get to his course. Then he sees Nick, a coach he knows, and bounces off to have a quick banter with him. Then he's back, and Teele and Matt are there, and he somehow isn't quite meeting my eye.

Right. Now Dan is sucking up to Matt Brears. Why? He's joking with him as if I didn't exist. I look at Teele, but she's gazing off into the distance. No one wants to talk to me, not even my mixed doubles partner. I feel like someone's mum. It seems that Matt and Teele play for the University of Kent First Team, but when I try to ask Dan about how he knows Matt, he ignores me. WTF? I feel like I've gone to youth club with my older brother and don't know what to say to fit in. Or worse, that this is my son and his friends and I am just completely invisible and irrelevant. It would be nice to have some banter with Dan myself because I'm actually quite anxious about this match. I've played with really good women before, but this will be the first time I've played competitively with a guy who's so strong.

We warm up with Teele whacking balls at my head at 300 miles per hour. I deal with it fine, but is it really necessary? She wins the warm-up, anyway, by about a bazillion points. We start playing. Dan serves first—his big, bold serve—and we win the game. This isn't so bad! Then it's Matt to serve, because the man always serves first, because the man is always better (except when Victoria Azarenka plays mixed and she goes on the ad side and serves first because she's better than her mixed partner, which I have always found so, so cool). I stand well back and prepare myself for the huge first serve I've seen in the warm-up, but instead I get a spinning second serve that completely throws me. I mean, I can't even get to it because I'm standing back so far. What the fuck? This little twat thinks I can't handle his first serve? Maybe he's right, but I'd like the chance to try. And surely if you're going to play a second serve out of kindness you should tell the person to expect it? Otherwise, maybe it isn't so kind after all.

Just this small act breaks me psychologically. They are all laughing at me. They all think I'm old, pathetic, rubbish. My serve is a joke compared with all theirs. Teele has an amazing but bizarre kicking first serve that goes so wide it's irretrievable. Dan gets annoyed because I can't return it. He suggests I stand out wider, but of course when I do that, she blasts one down the T. At least in this game I am not troubled by thoughts of winning. I don't even keep score. I try to make little in-jokes with Dan but I get nothing back, so I stop. Teele and Matt win 6–2, 6–0.

Our next opponents are Sara Fairclough—the one with the big topspin forehand and her own court in Sandwich and today wearing a yellow pleated Stella McCartney skirt I rather like—and Joseph Sevier, whom I have never met. Dan goes back to normal once Teele and Matt have gone and we start hitting together. He's making more mistakes than usual, though. He must be tired—turns out he actually got up at 4:00 a.m. to go to his Level 4 course. We agree that we'll take out whatever frustration we feel about Teele and Matt on Sara and Joseph. Dan says there's a trophy for coming second, which we will surely do. We take the first set comfortably enough, 6–4. I'm playing quite well, which is making up for some of the mistakes creeping into Dan's game. There are a lot of them.

In the next set, he completely falls apart. I haven't seen him implode quite so spectacularly before. Why is he doing this? These are beatable opponents, for goodness' sake. Don't we want that trophy? But Dan is on fire, and not in a good way. He serves double faults while going for ridiculous aces; hits the ball out or in the net when going for clear winners. At one of the changeovers I tell him we can win if he only puts 80 percent, or even less, into his shots. He carries on giving 120 percent. We lose the set. I can't take another championship tiebreak. Somehow we lose that too.

So that's it. I lost everything. Literally everything.

I go home and cry and drink wine. I look up Stella McCartney's current tennis clothes online, but I don't deserve any of it because I am a pathetic loser.

•

On Friday I go for my session with Josh, who is lovely and reassuring.

"I basically lost every single match," I admit to him. "I feel like a complete failure. I don't know what to do."

"You just need to play much more aggressively," he says.

This means taking the ball earlier, inside the baseline. It means continuing to try to get the elusive attacking forehand. With lots of topspin.

"Will I ever get it?" I ask. "I mean, should I just give up?"

I will get it, Josh says. But I have almost a year of bad habits to overcome.

"What you've done with Dan this last year," he says, grimacing. "I don't mean this to sound bad, but it has set you back. You'd have been better off not doing any of it, to be honest."

"Right."

"He's not even a good mixed partner for you, really. How late did he turn up this time?"

"Only ten minutes. But then he acted like a dick."

"You see?"

"I don't know why he has to show off all the time. We should have won against Sara and Joseph. It would have been easy."

"He's just holding you back," says Josh.

•

On Saturday I go to Walmer cricket ground to throw some balls down for Rod. He's nervous about playing cricket again after last year's shoulder operation and wants to practice his batting. Here, out in the open, in the bright green of the freshly mown pitch, I feel like an invalid. I can't bend my knees properly. Everything hurts when I run just a short distance to field the ball. I used to play cricket easily; now I can't. If I get down on the grass, it takes ages for me to get back up again, because I am just so stiff. I feel as if I am held together by rust. Can I do anything apart from play tennis?

The next day I go to the ITC to play with Lee. He is anxious because Liverpool looks like they are going to lose the Premier League. "You can be Liverpool," I say to him when we begin. "I'll be Man City." It's supposed to be a joke, but after I say it I feel like a bitch.

Anyway, after I beat him 6–2, 6–1, I do feel slightly better, but my lower legs are now like concrete. Later, at home, I stand in front of the mirror and properly look at my feet. My right foot barely has an arch but the left arch is so collapsed it looks ridiculous. I pull out the orthotics I hate so much. I'm not 100 percent sure why I hate them. Maybe it's because of all the barefoot running books I've read. After all, once you've got the primal/paleo thing down, then the next step is to sleep in the dark, then go barefoot, then go wild. This lifestyle appeals to me so much. Just before I did my ethnobotany course in 2010 I read *Guns, Germs, and Steel* by Jared Diamond. What a gripping, brilliant book! It confirmed what I have since read in all my paleo books: the agricultural revolution was a disaster for humanity. We'd have been better off—in health terms at least—by staying as hunter-gatherers.

Of course, then there'd be no poetry. No Shakespeare. No tennis.

I have to do something about my calves, though. Maybe the orthotics are the answer. Maybe civilization isn't so bad? I put them in my tennis shoes before going to Polo Farm the next evening for the mix-in session. Of course, you're supposed to build up to orthotics—start with five minutes, then ten, then fifteen. But does anyone really do that? I wear them for three hours straight, but it's only doubles on clay. By the end of the evening I'm becoming grumpy. I want to play beautiful, smooth, seamless, fast tennis. I want it to be transcendent and perfect and hard. But it takes me until about 9:00 p.m. to be put with the men's group I want to play with. I'm on with Richard, against Del and a guy I've never seen before named Dan. I serve an ace, which Dan calls out. Then he moans about my second serve being too shit.

"For fuck's sake," I say to Richard, a bit too loudly. "He doesn't want it fast, doesn't want it slow. Is he Goldilocks or something?"

Am I a little bit slower with the orthotics? Maybe slower is better than completely stopped due to cramp. Afterward I feel a bit worse in my right knee but a bit better everywhere else, except for the two new mosquito bites I suddenly seem to have on my left leg. I already have one on my right leg that is a bit red and swollen. I must remember insect repellent when playing outside in the evening, especially at Polo Farm, where the air is now a constant puff of rural smells and strange little insects.

Before I leave, Carol Bye comes over and asks me if I can play mixed doubles the following evening for Canterbury. It's in the East Kent league, and she's checked and I am eligible to play for Canterbury because I haven't yet played for the leisure center this season. All my matches have been in the Kent league, which is different.

"Sure," I say.

"Great. You're playing in Sandwich. You'll be with Nick Greenway. 7:00 p.m. start."

246 • SCARLETT THOMAS

•

The next day I have a coffee with Margaret. She wants to know about teams for the winter season, which confusingly starts in September. I say I want to play with Dan if possible, but I don't know what's happening with him and Hayley Palmer. Hayley doesn't even seem to like tennis that much anymore. On the way to Bearsted a few weeks before, we got chatting about it and she said she'd more or less given up on tennis. She said she preferred running, which you can do on your own, without all the gladiatorial pressure, the horrors of winning and losing. But she's somehow still on all the teams. That away match was the one we had to win to get into the league final, but I honestly now can't remember who won or lost. I just remember being scared of Hayley, and then leaving my quilted Barbour jacket behind in their changing rooms and never asking for it to be returned. I wonder where it is now.

Margaret and I chat about the French Open and gossip about the local leagues. I'd assumed Margaret was gay but in fact it turns out she is in love with Rafa. She even has a picture of him on her phone. Can you be gay and in love with Rafa? She starts telling me about all the times she's seen him at Wimbledon, how she once sat so close she got hit by a bead of his sweat when he shook his head near her.

"Have you got Wimbledon tickets?" she asks me.

"No."

"You didn't get any in our draw?"

"Nope."

"And not in Canterbury's?"

I shake my head.

"Well, do you want to come with me?" she asks. "I've got a spare ticket for the first Friday."

"Really?"

"Yes, we'll make a day of it. You'll have to bring sandwiches though. The way you do Wimbledon is you sit down in your seats and don't get up again for seven hours. It's the only way."

What about thrombosis? But I don't say this.

"Thank you," I say. "What do I owe you for the ticket?"

"Nothing. You can come as my guest."

•

I've bought a new gadget off Amazon. It's a little digital thingummy that you put on the end of your tennis racquet that gives you stats on your shots. You can find out whether you're hitting flat or with spin, how fast your serve is: all sorts of things. It turns out that the mystery woman I saw Dan with the other Sunday when I was playing with Hari is named Tatiana. He coaches her at Folkestone. Apparently she's too shy to play matches and always gets the yips on her serve. She also has one of these gadgets. In fact, Dan told me, you can set up a projector and see your stats in real time if you really want to. That's what Tatiana does sometimes. He says her name dreamily, with a little sigh afterward.

We have no projector, so I just play as well as I can for the session and resolve to look at my stats later once I've installed the right app on my iPhone. I love stats, so I can't wait.

In our drinks break I tell Dan I'm playing mixed for Canterbury tonight, against Sandwich. He's jealous, of course, but I point out that his mixed partner in this league is Hayley anyway, so.

"Right, well, I think that might change next season," he says. "I'm going to talk to Margaret."

"OK."

"I want to know *everything*," he says. "Who you play with, who you play against, the scores, literally everything."

"Sure."

For the rest of the session we play points. I'm level with Dan at five games all when Josh comes in. He's setting something up for his after-school kids' session, but he doesn't take his eyes off my shots. He doesn't do any of the embarrassing things that Dan does, like call out advice—and this isn't just because he's my secret coach. He even looks slightly impressed. I'm encouraged by his belief in me and so I manage to draw 6–6 with Dan by the time the session is over. As I leave, Josh gives me a little nod.

When I get home I can't wait to check out my stats, but they're disappointing. I'm not as fast as I thought, and even worse, all my forehands are deemed "flat." There isn't any sign of any topspin at all. What the fuck? Maybe the gadget is just broken, or wrong. It must be wrong. I package it up to return to Amazon.

At quarter to seven I arrive at the Sandwich tennis club. There are three macadam courts, two together and one on its own. There are portable toilets and lots of greenery. Even the birds seem to be green. Are those actual parakeets overhead, squawking in the dusk? They are. Sandwich is such a strange little town: a combination of super-rich golfers, international scientists, and the extremely elderly. Its proximity to Pfizer makes it feel more metropolitan than most small towns in the UK. Although Pfizer is closing down later this year, it's going to become a big science park.

Nick seems like a nice guy. Tall and lean with good focus. Probably a runner.

"What side do you want to play on?" he asks me.

I shrug. "I play both," I say.

"Which do you prefer?"

"Honestly? The ad side. But I usually play deuce in mixed, so."

He puts me on the ad side.

Our opponents are Phil and Bonita, and Stuart and Gemma. I recognize Stuart from the Canterbury Open. He was Lloyd Daniels's men's doubles partner. He's about my age, stocky, fit-looking, and friendly. At last, a couple of matches that I can win easily. It's not that these are bad players, they're not at all. But Gemma's rusty and Stuart is nervous and Nick is just the kind of steady doubles player I need. I'm getting to know some standard doubles plays now. The moonball over the head of the volleyer that draws the baseline player out wide. The sneaky shot down the tramlines. The whole thing is so enjoyable. I feel sorry for Sandwich, though. We win all our sets against them either 6–1 or 6–2.

The only problem is the mosquitos. I hadn't realized, but Sandwich, with its big river and all the greenery, is notorious for them. I keep reapplying repellent, but I'm not sure it's working. The main problem are the bites I got last week in Canterbury, which still seem a little bit itchy. After we finish playing I sit down on the wooden bench and text Dan. *We won!* I say. *I played on the ad side!!!*

Of course, he doesn't reply.

He definitely got the message, though.

In our session on Wednesday he has plenty to say about it.

"If I played against you and you were on the left I'd blast you with aces on your backhand side."

"Right."

"Why would this Nick guy want the lady on the left?"

"Maybe he's not a sexist dickhead?"

"I'd annihilate you if you played on the ad side against me."

"Yeah, you said that."

Today we work on serves. I'm given a basket of balls and told to practice throwing the ball higher, which is an issue for me. My throw is way too low. Dan videos me in secret and I think I'm watching a real tennis player for quite a few seconds before I realize that the athletic-looking woman with the amazing shoulder muscles on his phone is me. But he's still being weird about my match. He doesn't seem at all happy that I won. And this thing about me playing on the left has clearly bothered him. He keeps going on about it.

"If you had ten chances with this serve," I say. "You know, this ace that you say you'd blast me with if you encountered me on the ad side? How many do you think you'd get?"

"Ten," he says.

"OK," I say. "Let's do it."

Forty or so serves later he gives up. Of course the odds are in my favor. I know a big serve is coming, and I know it's going to be to my backhand. I hit some nice returns as well as edging and netting a few. But I get my racquet on all of them.

On Friday, Josh asks me where I think my level is, compared with Dan.

I shrug. Um and ah a bit.

"I think you're the same level," says Josh. "And soon you'll be better."

On Saturday, I wake up and find my body fat at under 30 percent for the first time in years. 29.8 percent! I want to run around with my knickers on my head. I feel so inspired. Are things finally starting to work at last? There's no tennis today, so I go off and have a great session in the gym. But that evening while Rod and I are watching the amazing women's final of the French Open, with Sharapova just edging it against Simona Halep with the most beautiful, powerful ground strokes, despite double-faulting all the time and looking like she might cry at any moment, my insect bites from last week start to really hurt. When I look, I see that these weird circles have developed around all three bites. All night my leg itches and burns. The next day I have a large, angry rash on my left ankle. In the *Guardian* the next day, Kevin Mitchell describes Sharapova's performance as the "vortex of suffering." My ankles feel a bit like that too.

On Sunday we have our next Aegon fixture, at home, against Tunbridge Wells Ladies. I'm playing with Margaret, and Hannah Martin is playing with Fiona. And of course we are all playing singles, too. I'm up first playing against a nice woman named Catherine Kirwen—Cathy—a fifty-year-old 9.1. Somehow, she's their highest-rated player, although apparently Sarah Luckhurst is pretty fearsome. Cathy's friendly and chatty, and I am too. I've completely dispensed with all of Brad Gilbert's advice.

Josh and the young assistant coach Adam have been playing a men's doubles, and they are having their afternoon tea right by where I'm playing. I do love an audience. I'm channeling Sharapova and thinking that if I am going to get beaten I'm going to do it in style, with my own vortex of suffering. Kind of dark, gothic, sexy tennis. Why not? Hannah and Fiona have been bagelled, or as good as, while Cathy and I have been wrapping up our first set, 6–3 to her. *Fuck it*, I think as we begin the second. *I've got nothing to lose. I'm going to go for the lines and hit as hard as I can.*

Cathy moves me around the court a lot, but I am fast and I am fit. She isn't going to break me down. In fact, I am possibly fitter than her? What happens if I move her around the court a bit? What happens if I just—yes—*blast* a ball down the line when she's not expecting it? We trade service games and then, on 2–2, I break her serve and then win mine. This is all it takes for me to go 4–2 up. Josh is leaving, but miming at me to text him my result. No one is expecting me to win, of course—no one here ever wins in Aegon singles, apart from Josh—but he wants to know the final result and how close it was.

Cathy wins the next game, so it's 4–3 to me. On the changeover she asks me where I got my skirt. It's actually the same one Simona Halep has been wearing in the French Open: it's purple, with orange shorts underneath. I'm wearing skirts with no leggings fine now, just like Halep and Sharapova. And although Halep is my favorite player on the tour this year, it's Sharapova that I continue to channel as Cathy and I go back on court. That beautiful, tragic desperation. Standing with my back to my opponent, looking at the black curtains, trying to compose myself before I serve. The only thing putting me off is that my insect bite rashes seem to have started to ooze green stuff. When I look more closely, it's tennis ball fluff stuck to the hydrocortisone cream I put on this morning. I win my service game.

I feel loose and relaxed. Aggressive, sharp. It's 5–4 to me and Cathy's serving. I am really going for it now: I blast my returns of serve past her and my balls kiss the lines hard and I keep thinking of Sharapova. I play every shot for a winner. Remarkably, many of them *are* winners. My grunt gets louder. The remaining men are sitting having their afternoon tea and if any of them glance over, I want them to see me fierce and strong and winning. I want them to hear me winning. I do little fist pumps. I turn my back on Cathy and check my strings before she serves. It's hot and I love it.

I win the second set 6–4.

As we go into the championship tiebreak, I am determined to keep my momentum going. It doesn't matter if I lose. Everyone else has lost. I don't at this point know Cathy's rating, but I assume it's higher than mine. The final score is another 10–8, but this time to me. To me! The first thing I do is call Rod, sweat and melted makeup dripping onto my iPhone, and tell him all about it. Then I text Josh. When I come back, it turns out Margaret has lost one and one to Sarah Luckhurst, even though her match seemed to be going on for a long time. She starts talking about all the deuces they had. Fiona and Hannah talk about their losses, how hard the opposition hit the ball, how we had no chance with them. They all look at me, and I realize that I am now supposed to say something about my loss, that I am supposed to complain about something too.

"I won my match," I say quietly.

"Sorry?" says Margaret.

"I won," I repeat. You *won*? they all say. It's the same when I give Margaret the score. I have to say it a couple of times before it sinks in that I did actually win my match. But I did. I won.

•

I've been playing a lot of tennis lately. So has Josh. On Monday morning we're both complaining about being knackered. It's 9:00 a.m. and we're still having sessions in secret.

"But at least we both won our matches," he says.

"Yeah."

We're talking about singles of course. In the doubles, Margaret and I lost love and one.

Josh's coaching sessions are hot and grueling. He feeds me balls that I hit down the line again and again and again. We do fast volleying sessions at the net.

"Next time can we maybe do two hours instead of one?" I say.

"Sure," says Josh.

One hour of tennis is just never enough for me now.

At around 9:45 a man comes in and starts warming up vigorously, running around in little circles and hitting a ball against a wall like something from a sketch show. He's clearly anxious to get on. He even helps pick up the balls from my session. I'm just getting my bag together to leave and I hear Josh saying, "You seem full of energy this morning, Graydon!" and Graydon saying back in a kind of North London drawl, "Yeah, that's because I didn't do any fucking drugs last night."

An hour later Josh texts me to say he's exhausted already: so much for starting the week so virtuously at 9:00 a.m. It's like having a friend. A normal one who actually remembers to text me. I really feel like an insider at the ITC now.

I'm off to work to do some admin and I stop at the Canterbury Sainsbury's on the way in. They have a good pharmacy there, and I'm far too busy to go to the doctor. My rash is now very red and very big and has started up on the other leg too, around the other mosquito bite. It's itching and burning like wildfire. I can't touch it. I feel a bit ill, too. The pharmacist says it's a fungal infection caused by the mosquito perhaps having been on a cow pat or something equally gross just before landing on me. He gives me cream and antihistamines, but by the end of the day I feel so bad I don't even consider going to tennis. When I try to imagine throwing a ball up above my head and then hitting it across the net, I just can't do it. I feel so exhausted all of a sudden. I go home and have a terrible night's sleep with my legs hanging out of the bed. They are so very hot, and so very itchy. It really is as if they are on fire.

Awake in bed, I keep thinking about my win against Cathy. I find myself haunted by a feeling that I didn't really win, that it was a mistake. It was very close, after all. Did I cheat? That wide serve she did on the ad side. It was out, and I called it out, but what if it was in? What if I saw it wrong? Since I won on a tiebreaker, there were only two points in it. Does that mean if I made two wrong line calls in the match that I didn't really win it? Then again, she called some close ones out too. There was the point we had to replay because she wasn't sure, but I was: I knew my shot was in.

I thought it would be great to finally be able to tell people that I have won something, but it turns out that most people are more interested in loss. I guess that's what I teach all the time: how much more drama there is in suffering, how no stories are happy. Who wants to read about happy characters? And telling happy stories isn't as much fun either.

•

On Tuesday I cancel Pilates and tennis and go back to Canterbury in search of my old homeopath Elaine, whom I haven't seen for a long time. I can't concentrate on anything at all, so I go in much earlier than I have to and walk around Fenwick, my favorite local department store, feeling like a zombie. I wonder if I'll be asked to leave because my legs look so dreadful. I hadn't intended to try anything on, and I can't bear the thought of anything going near my leg, but there is quite a nice dress that would only involve me removing the top half of what I'm wearing. OMG. I *have* lost weight. In the changing room mirror I see an athletic-looking woman with really a very nice bum, firm or firm-ish in places that were not firm before. I realize for the first time that although on the scales I have moved what seems only very slightly from around 153 lbs. to 149 lbs. (give or take) and from around 34 percent body fat to just under 30 percent, my body shape really is changing. I am so happy I even forget the burning in my legs for about two minutes. In the end I don't buy the dress, but because of it, not me.

Elaine doesn't like the look of my rash. She thinks it's cellulitis, a serious bacterial infection of the skin and the tissue beneath the skin. Unusually for a homeopath, she tells me to go to the ER or urgent care immediately. It's now too late for the trial and error sometimes needed to get the correct homeopathic remedy. I almost certainly need antibiotics before this gets even worse, before I end up in the hospital. All this from three little mosquito bites.

When I get to urgent care, I explain what happened to a nurse who can't believe it, has never seen anything like this before. She calls in another nurse—the one who gave me the dressing for my toe months ago. She's dyed her hair blonde. Neither of them know what it could be. Spiders, maybe? The town has apparently had an infestation of false widows in the last few years. But isn't it too early for spiders? Anyway, I was out in the open, not rooting around in a basement or a shed.

The nurses admire the patterns formed by the rash. On the left leg in particular the rash has formed something like a ring around the original bite, as if it were a tornado or crop circle. And it's spreading by the minute, down my leg toward my ankle. On my right leg the crop circles have merged and my skin is becoming more and more purple and swollen. They don't have a doctor at urgent care, so I'm sent down the hill to a GP who gives me antibiotics, strong steroid cream, and two types of antihistamine. What if these don't work? Then it's the hospital, for an antibiotic drip. But they do work, and quite quickly. By the next morning the itching has reduced and by the afternoon it is gone. But the ghost of the rash will stay on my legs for weeks. Perhaps it's all a coincidence, but I won't feel quite right again for almost three years.

9

Nottingham

A tennis court is a rectangle seventy-eight feet long and thirty-six feet wide. The service line is twenty-one feet from the net. The net is three feet six inches high at the posts and three feet at the center. It does not adhere to the principle of the Golden Ratio exactly, but has the same feel: the beauty, rightness, and calm of the rectangular box, in which drama and struggles take place, and people win and lose and triumph and fail, but in which you can also hide from life indefinitely, safe within the invisible four walls, surrounded by netting.

•

When I go down for my next session with Josh, he's finishing what looks like a session on serving with Lucille. There's a life-size cardboard cutout of Andy Murray standing in the receiver's position in the opposite deuce court, which is not where it should be. Andy had to be moved down to the tennis center after the lifeguards and reception staff upstairs abused him so badly that his head had to be stapled back on to his body. But now he's down here, people just hit balls at him until he falls over.

"I'll tell Dan on you," I say once Lucille has gone. Dan is very protective of Andy.

It's a good session with Josh. My legs are almost completely better and my knees are responding to all the green-lipped mussel extract I've thrown at them, and all the foam-rolling I am now doing. I can chase down balls better and move more freely into my forehands and backhands. My topspin forehand is finally making sense. But I'm still having trouble with the drive volley. "Trust your strings," says Josh. "You have the best strings in the world. Trust them." The idea is to play across the ball horizontally with the racquet facing the same way throughout, just like a topspin forehand, but higher and with—seemingly—less pushing into the shot. After I fluff lots of them, Josh has a brainwave. "Try hitting *up*," he says. This makes no sense. The ball is high and I want to bring it down into the court so I should hit down, right? But I do what he says and suddenly that's it, that's the shot. He jumps out of the way. "You hit that pretty hard!" he says. I do two more and then my brain freezes again and I can't do it. This is the point where Dan would make me carry on, perhaps tying my arm to something or covering my racquet in a carrier bag. But we simply move on to the backhand for a while. It'll come back, Josh says. But when?

Afterward we sit and chat. Josh is happy because he's just got the wins he needs to go up to a 3.1. I'm still pleased with my victory over Cathy, but now I need ratings wins. And of course it would be nice to win a prestigious local tournament.

"Are you excited for the Walmer Open?" Josh asks.

"Yeah. I think so. A bit nervous."

"Well, it looks like Lucille won't be playing. That'll open up the draw for you."

"Why isn't Lucille playing?"

"She's been called up to play for the county over-35s and they have a match that week."

"Oh. Right."

"Yeah, apparently she beat someone—Karen or Corrine Cross or something—"

"Kerrin Cross."

"Yeah, at the Spring Open. And Kerrin Cross plays for the county. She's sixth in the country for over-35s or something."

"Yeah."

"And Lucille's been playing Aegon for Canterbury, of course."

Stuff goes through my head. I'm playing for Canterbury too! But not Aegon. I start to tell Josh about Sue Depledge and how a friend of mine who I almost beat almost beat her in the Canterbury tournament and how Sue's tenth in the country for over-35s but the standard isn't so high and that actually I could probably beat her or at least come close—

"Really?" Josh says, disbelievingly. He realizes how incredulous his tone is and says it again in a more neutral way, but the damage is done. We both laugh but I do feel a bit crushed. But then, what do I really expect? I can't even hit a decent topspin backhand consistently yet. I lose most of my matches. I still have not mastered the drive volley I want so much or, of course, the high topspin forehand with which high-rated players annihilate low-rated players and which low-rated players need if they are to become high-rated players.

"I guess Lucille is really good," I say. "Didn't she play in South Africa?"

"She was in the top ten under-18s. She still hits the ball very nicely. I'd love to have seen her playing then."

•

On Sunday I'm meeting my good friend Gonzalo at Polo Farm for a game. Gonzalo is Chilean. His family is in no way poor, but he is always struggling with visa issues and the awful policies of our ever more racist government. He did his undergraduate degree at Kent, then got a distinction in his MA in postcolonial studies, and then did the Contemporary Novel PhD program with me. He's currently in an extension year trying to find a job that will give him Tier 2 visa sponsorship. If he can't get it, he'll have to go back to Santiago, where he hasn't lived since he was a kid. He's super-stressed trying to work all this out but never shows it. He turns up at Polo Farm in a cool band T-shirt and skater shorts. A large bandage covers a new tattoo he's just had done.

How strange it is to step outside the tennis bubble I've been in and play someone "normal." I know my serve is OK and I can win points off it when I need to, but it is quite thrilling to see a fit and healthy twenty-seven-year-old guy unable to return it at all.

"Oh my God, Scarlett," Gonzalo says. "Your serve is monstrous."

I hit an ace down the T that shoots off the line. Out of politeness I ask Gonzalo if it was in.

"I don't know, man," he says. "It was so fast I didn't even fricking see it."

We play the point again. As we play I notice something. I am beginning to be able to generate my own pace on the ball. That time I played Hari, my serve looked good but I struggled to play proper ground strokes off his slower balls. Here, I decided early that I'd just practice perfecting my topspin, rolling the ball over the net in that delicious way I now can. I do this down the line a few times and although it doesn't feel like I am putting tons of power behind the shot, the topspin is what has the effect and the ball shoots off the court toward the back fence.

"Oh my God, Scarlett," Gonzalo says again. "How am I even supposed to get to that?" I do it again. "That's beautiful, man."

•

On Wednesday, I play Paul Gregory in the Canterbury LTC box leagues, one of the reasons I joined Canterbury. You are put in a "box" with three other players and everyone in the box plays everyone else. It's always singles, and is genderless—men can play women. The other exciting thing is that the matches count for ratings.

It's taken a while to set up this game. I had to cancel our first arranged fixture because of my skin infection. Then Paul canceled the alternative because neither of us had realized we'd scheduled our game against England's first match in the World Cup. Now here we are. It's a beautiful sunny day with a touch of wind. I hadn't been sure how to picture Paul from his texts, but he turns out to be a tall, athletic-looking man of around my age. We joke that today we are both "working from home," and in fact he really does have a conference call to get back for later. I suppose I might write a paragraph or two for my tennis book.

We start knocking up and it is immediately clear that this man is coached. He has a nice contemporary style. Plenty of topspin, playing the ball early. Am I going to lose this? He's a 10.2, which we all know means nothing, but I really, really don't want a ratings loss here. He hits the ball hard. His volleys are crisp and clean.

We spin for the serve and he wins.

A 6–0 set is a curious thing. It moves so fast that it isn't exactly clear who is doing what to whom, or even why one person is being so completely crushed by the other. I'm not sure how I do it, but I do take the first set 6–0. Paul hits the ball hard, but it often goes out.

He double-faults. But it's not just that he plays erratically and I play steadily; I hit a lot of actual aggressive winners myself.

During the second set Paul follows a weak approach shot into the net and I lob him: it's a beautiful looping topspin forehand that circles over and over itself before falling just on the baseline and then hurling itself into the back netting. I'm so busy watching the ball that I don't realize Paul has fallen over. He's lost the ball in the sun and his footing with it.

"You OK?" I ask.

"Yeah," he says, picking himself up. "Just a graze."

A couple of points later, he comes in off the same approach shot. He's still into the sun. I still lob him.

"I see you went for the lob again," he says on the changeover.

"I mean, you did come into the net," I say.

I win the second set 6–0 as well. While we're packing up afterward, Del walks past the netting.

"You win?" he says to me. I nod.

"Love and love," I can't help saying, even though Paul is listening.

Chatting to Paul while packing up, I discover that Nicholas Handley, the only other player in our box since Fin Murray said he was too busy to play, beat Paul 6–0, 6–0. And just like that my victory loses its sweetness, like a bruised section of an otherwise juicy peach. Paul asks me when I'm playing Nicholas, but it's been even harder to arrange that game.

In Nicholas's first text to me he said that as he has "a young family" he can only play on Sunday mornings. Could I play at 9:00 a.m.? Was he joking? I texted back that the very, very earliest I could play on a Sunday—a *Sunday!*—would be 10:00 a.m. Even then, I was thinking he'd almost certainly thrash me because it'd be so early and I'd be a little hungover. I could of course just not drink on Saturday night, but who does that? I relay some of this to Paul.

"I played him at 7:00 a.m.," he says, as if that's normal.

Good lord.

Paul hurries away for his conference call. I sit by the clubhouse drinking water and watching Tiegan Aitken. She's being coached by Simon as usual, but someone else is there, serving at her. Maybe a parent? Tiegan is upset after fluffing a shot and she's having a bit of a tantrum.

"Never let them see it," the parent is saying. "Never let anyone see they've hurt you. Never give them the satisfaction of getting to you. So what do we put on? A neutral face. And what does a neutral face look like?"

Tiegan slams her racquet into the fence.

"No, Tiegs, it doesn't look like that. Can you do me a neutral face?"

She's scowling now. Crying. Hiding her face in her towel.

"Please?" says the parent.

Simon's collecting balls near where I'm sitting. He comes over to me.

"Is everything OK?" he asks. "I saw what happened in your match."

"I know," I say, beaming. "I won love and love."

"No," he says. "I mean Paul. I saw him fall. Is he OK?"

"Er, yeah, I think so."

"I saw you lob him again when he was facing the sun."

"He was the one who came in off a bad approach shot."

Simon walks off, unimpressed.

•

It's the First Friday of Wimbledon and I'm meeting Margaret on the 8:11 train from Ramsgate. We'll arrive at Victoria and then take the Tube to Southfields, from which it is a brisk fifteen-minute walk to the stadium. I'm a little bit afraid of crowds and terrorism and so on, but fuck it, I really want to go and see some live tennis.

I've packed gluten-free rolls with vegan sausages and mustard in them. At the moment I'm trying not to eat dairy, because I think this will help me lose more fat. I'm worried about spending all day sitting on my arse eating, though. I'm looking forward to watching tennis, but I'd much, much rather be playing.

On the train there, Margaret and I talk constantly. We talk about the players on the Herne Bay team, and why they always seem to win. Is Margaret ever going to stop playing for Herne Bay? We laugh about the time I went to play there in high winds when the only doubles partner available for the leisure center was Kofo and Margaret and her partner beat us love and love. Haha! Margaret talks about how reliable Josh is, and how Dan really needs to buck his ideas up and pass his Level 4 or else what exactly is the point of him? Poor Dan. I bring up the thing about Lucille being selected to play for the county. I talk about Kerrin Cross and Sue Depledge and the county rankings. I've become a bit of a nerd about the rankings.

"Oh God," says Margaret, dismissively. "Those women aren't really the top ten players in Kent. Everyone knows those rankings don't mean anything. No one's even heard of those players."

"Really?"

"You want the best players in Kent, you're looking at the real county players. People like Sarah Luckhurst, Sue Boffey. You won't see them in the county rankings."

"Is that because they mainly play doubles, though?" I say. "What about singles?"

Margaret gives me an intense kind of look.

"When you reach a certain age," she says. "It really is all about doubles."

"Right."

"Although of course county matches do have singles as well, I think in the over-40s as well as the over-35s. But you've got to be a very strong player to even be considered."

Wimbledon—the All England Lawn Tennis and Croquet Club—is not at all what I expected. I've been brought up to be suspicious of big events that might catch fire or blow up or at the very least have wasps and long queues. As a family we simply never did the uncool, sheep-like things that normal people would consider a good time. Our idea of a good Saturday afternoon out was a trip to the alternative bookstore Compendium Books in Camden, or Dillon's in Cambridge, where if I was lucky someone would buy me a terrifying book about children surviving nuclear war but then getting cancer and dying. We did stately homes and the occasional woodland walk. My mother went through a long phase of wanting to go and find forgotten women's graves. I remember the pain of the stinging nettles as we hacked through the undergrowth toward Sylvia Plath's headstone on a holiday in Yorkshire when I was fifteen.

But this is so nice! Wimbledon is airy, happy, light. People are actually having fun. Our tickets are for Court 2 and so we walk by the entrance to Centre Court and past the small show courts before we present our tickets to the officials. We sit there all day, four rows up, with a great view, watching every match that takes place. We miss the very start of Simona Halep against Lesia Tsurenko, which Simona wins 6–3, 4–6, 6–4. I love her style of play: aggressive and sleek. She is so strong and beautiful. She is exactly the same height as me. She wears Adidas and has a Wilson racquet, like me.

Margaret warned me on the train that watching "real" tennis was going to be a shock, because "real" players hit it so much harder and faster than we amateurs. But I am surprised to see that the tennis I'm watching is actually not that much different from the tennis I play. Am I deluding myself? Almost certainly. But there is something tantalizing about the fact that what we do recreationally is so close to what the pros do. We don't do it quite as hard and fast, but we play the same length matches, in the same size rectangle, and with the same range of shots.

We watch a very long five-set game between Jerzy Janowicz and Lleyton Hewitt. At some point it rains briefly and we go to the gift shop, where Margaret opens a coffee table book of photographs and shows me a picture of herself sitting behind the scoreboard on Court 1 during one of Rafa's matches.

Toward the end of the day we get large glasses of white wine and sit there in the evening sunshine as planes trail their white vapor behind them and birds fly lazily overhead. Super-skinny Agnieszka Radwańska has beaten Michelle Larcher de Brito 6–2, 6–0, and the final match of the day is a men's doubles with Jamie Murray and some other dudes. I don't really care about the tennis anymore. I'm just soaking up the lovely end-of-day vibes.

On the way back, we walk past the last matches being played on the unticketed courts. There are a couple of junior matches taking place. Barely anyone is in the audience, maybe twenty people watching each one. I think about Tiegan Aitken, and how many hours, days, weeks, and months of sheer hard work it would take her to get here. But once you're here, no one really cares unless you're one of the big names. You could be everything in your local club and nothing here. Apparently, minor WTA matches don't get any audience at all. You could get to within the top fifty players in the world and you could play a match and still no one would care.

•

Inspired by Wimbledon, I have a quick ball machine session the next day. I feel amazing and inspired and light on my feet. But then Rod and I are off for a weekend with friends in London. I now can't bear being without tennis for even two days. Make that one and a half, because I'm playing with Josh on Monday morning before I go to Devon to spend a few days with Mum and Couze.

Our friends Denis and Mary are lovely, and conversation is great, but I realize how much I feel like a child in these situations at the moment, wanting to jiggle and scratch and go and run around outside. At the height of my absorption with alcohol and food, I remember thinking about how great it was to not be a child anymore. As a child I was bored by dinner parties or Sunday lunches with the grown-ups. I could barely manage one course when we ate out, and never ordered pudding. Being a grown-up so far has meant drinking a lot and eating a lot and being very clever and saying outrageous things. Surely any child would want that, rather than the empty boredom of a Sunday afternoon with no sauvignon blanc or Picpoul to look forward to. But I've come full circle and I would genuinely now rather be at the gym, rowing back and forth, listening to Chiddy Bang, and preparing myself for tennis. I don't even really like the feeling of being full and drunk anymore, especially not compared with the feeling of being fit and strong. It's just taken a very long time to get here, and if I didn't love tennis so much I would never have even begun the journey.

•

On Monday morning I turn up for my 9:00 a.m. session with Josh a few minutes early as usual. As soon as I open the double doors into the ITC I know something's wrong. Dan's unmistakable blue Head bag is lying there just outside the office. Fuck. Dan is never up by 9:00 a.m., let alone in the ITC. And he doesn't come in until after lunch on Monday anyway, because he stays until 9:00 or 10:00 p.m.

Josh comes out of the office and gives me an *oh, fuck* look. Then he adds a barely perceptible little smile, like it's an oh-fuck situation he's actually going to enjoy.

It's too late. We can't hide what we're doing. We slope off to Court 4 and close all the netting and sort of pretend we're invisible—well, I do. Josh seems entirely unashamed. He does everything he can to make it obvious from a distance that I'm being coached, like standing on the same side of the net as me and feeding me balls from baskets. Graydon has the 10:00 a.m. slot as usual and so we chat for a couple of minutes while Josh goes to the office for something.

"You beaten him yet?" asks Graydon.

"What, Josh?" I laugh. "Yeah. Haha."

"I've taken a few games off him."

"Right." I gather up my stuff. "You're an actor, Josh said?"

"Yeah. And a screenwriter. Fucking brutal life."

"Mm. I'm a novelist myself. Try and keep out of the world of screens."

"You had anything published?"

"Er, yeah. Quite a lot."

"You want to have a hit sometime?"

I shrug. "Yeah, sure."

As long as this conversation continues, I don't have to face Dan. But soon Josh comes back and I have to do the walk of shame across Courts 3, 2, 1. Dan is sitting at one of the round tables by the notice boards looking sad.

"You all right?" I say.

"Yeah," he says. "How was your coaching with Josh?"

"Um, good," I say. "Of course, you know I like hitting with you best, right?"

He nods. Doesn't meet my eye. His head droops a bit.

I don't really know what to do. "So . . ."

He suddenly snaps back into being Dan. "Tomorrow 2:00 p.m.!" he says brightly.

"Oh, no, actually. Remember I said I was going to Devon?"

"Oh." He sips some of his drink. "You gonna go to a local mix-in? I could come too? Imagine that. We could turn up and kill everyone at doubles, bang, bang, bang!"

"What, you'd come to Devon?"

"I was going to move there once. Did I ever tell you about that?"

"Where?"

"Totnes."

"That's where I'm going!"

"Cool!"

"OK, but my mother has banned me from bringing my tennis racquet. I'm not sure what she'd say about me bringing my tennis coach."

"Hitting partner."

"What?"

"And friend. Josh's your coach now. It's OK."

•

In Devon I dream of tennis, as usual. Most nights I am plowing my way through some tournament or other. As I fall asleep I am hitting forehands over and over, perfect topspin winners down the line, crosscourt, and inside out. Up and over, up and over, until blackness takes over.

It's the second week of Wimbledon. Yesterday we—Mum, Couze, and I—watched both Sharapova and Nadal crash out, then much of the Kvitová match was taken up with my mother describing to me how Couze recently managed to set fire to the salad drawer from the fridge. At some point I nipped out to the local gym and did a couple of circuits, some rowing intervals, and some experiments with a medicine ball.

Last night I dreamed of tennis as usual until something spooked me and I had to spend the rest of the night with a lamp switched on.

There's a lot of tennis to watch today.

"I have watched tennis all my life," says my mother mysteriously, before disappearing to her study to smoke and write reports on her psychotherapy clients.

I've been struck on this visit by how hard Mum and Couze still work, even though Mum's sixty-six and Couze is in his seventies. Mum has all her clients, with their notes and emails and phone calls, and Couze has recently taken on a heavy workload at Goldsmiths, teaching an MA course and supervising various PhD students. He does it all much more thoroughly than me. He even speaks to his students on the phone. As well as all this, he is also on the editorial board for the journal *Theory, Culture & Society*. He had a Skype with his other editors on the morning before I arrived that went on for five and a half hours. I can't remember the last time I did anything for five and a half hours, certainly not work. People see me as incredibly productive and an extremely hard worker, but what do I actually do all day? I drift around thinking about tennis, playing tennis, training for tennis, or doing things connected with tennis.

I still have a slight addiction to buying new stuff which I wish I could overcome. Yesterday I spent the morning in Totnes waiting for Mum to finish seeing clients and meet me for lunch. I bought two jackets, a pair of jeans, two T-shirts, and a dress. Having this new body is not helping in this respect. Stuff looks nice when I try it on and then I buy it. Even this morning, watching Simona Halep playing Sabine Lisicki, a part of me is coveting Simona's white, skater-style Adidas skirt. I already have approximately £250 worth of Simona's skirts. I also have her visors: the purple one and the white one.

My mother comes in. "Which one's that?" she asks.

"Lisicki," I say. "She was the finalist last year."

"Your legs are nicer than hers," Mum says.

She goes to the kitchen and makes a cup of tea and then comes back and starts reading the *Daily Mirror*.

"Did I mention that you were born during Wimbledon?"

"Yes."

"You were a Wimbledon baby."

"I know."

Simona Halep plays an amazing second set, beating Lisicki in the end 6–4, 6–0. She is so strong and beautiful. Her hair is so shiny. Apparently she had breast reduction surgery to improve her tennis, which certainly captured the imagination of many of the aging perverts who follow the WTA Tour. Once she has finished celebrating, I switch over to find Eugenie Bouchard on the verge of beating Angelique Kerber.

"Your legs are nicer than hers, too," says Mum.

Then it's time for Andy Murray to play Grigor Dimitrov.

"I can't watch," says Mum, putting the *Daily Mirror* away.

Dimitrov serves first. Mum is howling before the first point is over. When Murray nets the ball she lets out a painful yelp. The next time, another one.

"He always does this."

"Mmm."

"I've always said. He always does this on that shot."

"Mum, we're like two points into the match."

"Judy needs to give him a good talking-to. Or maybe what's her name? That new female coach?"

"Amelie Mauresmo."

"Or Kim. I do like her hair. ANDY!"

"He's not really expected to break serve in the first game. Give him a chance."

But poor Murray doesn't really get any energy flowing at all and before long he's trailing badly in the first set. Couze goes out to do some gardening.

"I told you so," says Mum. "I can't bear it. You see that weird man in the cowboy hat? I'm going to google him instead."

She gets out her iPad. I can't really complain. While Rafa was being beaten I was occasionally googling images of toenail fungus.

"See! I told you he was someone." Mum waves her iPad at me, but I don't really look.

Andy nets another ball.

"He needs his little bottom smacked."

"Mum!"

"If he was my son I'd tell him, 'You're not too old to go over my knee.'"

"That's seriously disgusting."

"Hmm. I prefer Kim's hair to Kate Middleton's."

"Yeah." I can at least concede this.

"Do you think William chose the wrong one?"

I give Mum a vaguely WTF look. The players are on a change-over. The camera lingers on a retired rugby player.

"Why is it," Mum says, "that the most disgusting, ugly, old sportsmen get the most beautiful young wives?" I don't respond.

"Are you ignoring me?"

"I'm blocking you out."

"What are you writing?"

"I'm writing down all the ridiculous things you are saying so I can put them in my book."

"No! That's so embarrassing!"

"If you think it's too embarrassing to go in my book then it's probably too embarrassing to say."

After Dimitrov wins the match, and once Mum has gone back to the *Daily Mirror*, I start browsing seniors' tournaments on the LTA site. Here's a Grade 1 national seniors' tournament. Grade 1. Frightening, and completely out of my league if it weren't a seniors' tournament, which it is, but it's at the All England Club. Isn't that— hang on, that's Wimbledon! There is a seniors' tournament at Wimbledon. At the end of August. And it's open for entries now.

Above each tournament description on the LTA site is a word or two that tells you its category. British Tour; County Closed; Regional Tour; Match Play; Seniors. Most of the time the category doesn't mean that much, unless it is County Closed, in which case you have to be from the right county to enter. Above the All England Club British Seniors Grass Court Championships entry, all it says is CLOSED. So that's that then. Closed must surely mean Closed to the likes of me. Perhaps you have to be a member of the All England Club to play. It's not clear. But for some reason I put the tournament on my watchlist anyway.

No one has yet entered the women's singles over-35 or over-40 categories, but men are starting to enter in their age groups. I scrutinize some of these men. They seem to come from all over the country. There's a 2.2 from Cheshire who is the current national over-40s champion. But there's also a 9.2 from Middlesex with an average-to-good club player's profile. I read the terms and conditions for the tournament but it doesn't say anything about what "Closed" means. Eventually I think, *Fuck it.* I'm a novelist, I do embarrassing and awkward things for a living. I'll just enter the tournament and then if it's closed to me presumably someone will realize and throw me out. I got expelled from school. It was fine. I can be expelled from Wimbledon. I can take it. And it might make a funny little episode in my tennis book. It costs £38. And this is to *play* at Wimbledon. If you want to go and *watch* tennis at Wimbledon it costs £56 and involves a series of complex raffles and ballots that begin the previous September. This is awesome. Well, it will be until they throw me out.

•

Of course, I did bring my tennis racquet. It's a lovely warm evening in Totnes. Around twelve people have come for the club night. It's a great idea, to let visitors and would-be new members pay £5 per session. Last time I came to one of these sessions was that disastrous evening last September, when I didn't know which side I should stand on or what I should do. I remember a woman, so frustrated, hissing at me to "cover the tramlines." I was hungover, sad, in pain. No one wanted to play with me. I lost every single game I played.

Today I warm up in the gym. After I've finished, the fit-looking guy from the office follows me out and at first I think it's to check that I did my induction or something, but in fact he's seen me row-ing and wants to know if I'm interested in joining his indoor rowing team. Perhaps he does this to everyone? But I know I'm a good rower so I allow myself to feel a bit chuffed and go over to the tennis courts feeling happy and excited. This time it will be different. I feel so at home now on a tennis court, in a tennis club, calling *van in* and *van out* and making guys try to ace me because it's the only way they can be sure of a point on their serve.

Although suffering makes for a good narrative, for the next two hours there simply isn't any. I feel at home with tennis people, on a tennis court. I know where to stand, what to do. I chat happily about Roger and Stan's quarterfinal—the Swiss derby—and what a shame it is about Andy but how well Dimitrov did to beat him. I'm still not the world's greatest doubles player, but these people take me seriously. I am one of them. I belong.

•

I'm signed up to play a seniors' tournament in Nottingham beginning on July 16. Two events: ladies' over-30 singles and ladies' over-40 singles. At one point there were seven in the over-30 and four in the over-40 but suddenly Sue Depledge dropped out of both. Then someone else withdrew from the over-40. Then the organizer sent around an email suggesting that the two events merge. Then he did the draw and it turns out that I'm up first against the number 2 seed, a 5.2 who would have had a bye in the original lineup, leaving me to play an 8.1 in the first round. There is no compulsory conso-lation draw.

Since the over-40 singles was going to be played as a round robin, I have gone from a potential four or five guaranteed matches to only one. I have suggested that Lynn, the other over-40, and I still play our match, which I guess will be classed as a Grade 3 final. The organizer says that yes, we can do this, as long as we can find a convenient time and a court. Lynn is on the same side of the main draw as me in the over-30, which makes things look unnecessarily complicated. I could end up playing her twice. Or not at all. This is becoming too flaky.

I ask the organizer about the consolation draw and he says he'll run one but can't guarantee that others will enter it. I don't really want to spend hundreds of pounds going to Nottingham to get beaten by a 5.2 and then stress about other matches that are not definite. I do want to be beating 5.2s in the nearish future, but I know I'm not ready yet. And of course I'd like an easy stab at a Grade 3 final, but even if I won it would feel a bit like I got the ranking points by slightly foul means. I'd go up in the Kent rankings beyond Lucille and into the top five, but it would not mean I'm better than her. It would not mean I am a county player. It would just mean I got lucky with math. On the Totnes-Paddington train I email the organizer to say I am pulling out, but we've barely reached Exeter before I have a change of heart and email him to say I'm back in again—as long as I can definitely play Lynn.

So I'm going to go to Nottingham on the cheap. Well, still First Class, obviously, although the advance tickets are only £21 each way. I know when I'm going but not when I am coming back, but I book my ticket for the afternoon of the final. And I seem to have found a £50-a-night hotel with a sauna, steam room, and pool. I am almost certain the pool will have dead bodies floating in it. I mean, £50 a night! But still, an adventure for the book and all that.

•

It's my birthday on July 5, women's finals day—I was a Wimbledon baby, as my mother is always pointing out. But I feel low the day before and low on my birthday. I can never think of anything I really want to do on my birthday. Last year Rod and I went for a macrobiotic picnic in Goodnestone Park Gardens and I thought about buying myself a tennis coaching session. The year before was my fortieth, which I spent feeling fragile and hungover at the Damian Hirst exhibition at the Tate Modern, watching flies buzzing around a rotting cow's head. The year before, 2011, was when my brother Sam and I were in touch with Steve Sparkes again for the first time in over twenty-five years, but he was dying and, far closer to home, my beloved dog Dreamer was dying, and by the end of July it was all over. Sam and I never quite recovered from having to clean all the syringes out of Steve's awful flat, and I found I just couldn't get over Dreamer's death, no matter how hard I tried. July always makes me sad now.

Each year I wonder if my father Gordian will get in touch on my birthday. Sometimes he does; more often he doesn't. When I was a kid and it was still a secret about him being my father, he always bought me the best presents: one year a real Walkman, another year a massive expensive stereo. I told my school friends that he was my uncle/godfather and they thought I was lying because I could never get my story straight. I told everyone that my uncle/godfather was the manager of OMD but no one I knew liked OMD.

This year, he doesn't get in touch.

Should I have texted him on his birthday in April? But to say what? All I want him to do is get in his car and come and see me here in Kent where I live in a beautiful house with my lovely partner. But he won't and I don't know why. At Steve's funeral, Gordian talked about how his daughter Katherine had been talking all the time on holiday about wanting to see her sister: me. I want this too. Why can't it just happen? But it never seems to. Is it because I'm not trying hard enough? Gordian's not trying at all, but he's neurotic and depressed and maybe therefore it's up to me.

I must try harder. At everything.

The only thing I really want to do on my birthday is play tennis, but I have no one to play with. Dan and the rest of the mixed doubles team are in Gravesham, a long way across Kent, for an away fixture that I didn't fancy playing on my birthday. So I end up at the leisure center with the ball machine. I can't even hide away on Court 4 because our men's team are playing Canterbury, which means that Lee is there, and Jon Wise, and Paul Gregory. Instead I have to go on Court 1, the most public court. I put my headphones on and turn Chiddy Bang up loud and ignore everyone.

For no definite reason I feel on the verge of tears the whole time I'm playing. I can't get my backhand to go right. My forehand is so much better, but why isn't it perfect? The ball machine sends a couple of balls short and I naturally use them as approach shots. I think I might practice some volleys, but I'm not that close to the net and— OMG. I just hit a drive volley! A real one, my racquet swishing through the air like a knife spreading butter. The ball machine spits out another ball and I try it again. Bang! The ball hits the baseline with so much force and topspin that it thwacks into the curtain with all the certainty of a definite winner. Quite a frightening winner. The next ball comes and I do it again. The next one I fluff. But over the rest of the session I hit so many drive volleys that when I finish my little finger is bleeding.

Rod's brother Murray is here from Auckland, so we go out for dinner for my birthday and talk about tennis and books. Then we come home a bit drunk and watch Petra Kvitová thrash Eugenie

Bouchard. It's a beautiful, brutal game, made more pleasurable by how big-headed Bouchard was going into it, and how much she deserved to lose. The whole thing only takes fifty-five minutes.

On Sunday morning, Graydon texts to see if I want to play tennis later. I would have done, perhaps, but I've already been to the gym and am looking forward to flopping out in front of the men's final all afternoon. I text him back that I'm planning to nurse my hangover in front of the tennis, which sounds a bit better than admitting to already having been to the gym. He texts back, *You sound like a lager lout.* I suggest playing on Thursday but he replies that he can't plan anything that far ahead because he might get called for an audition. We agree to confirm on Wednesday.

On Monday night I manage to have a bit of a meltdown at the mix-in at Polo Farm. Judith has finished reading one of my novels. I'd recommended *The End of Mr. Y*, which everyone likes, but she's read *Our Tragic Universe*, which only hard-core fans really love.

"To be honest," she says, "and don't take this the wrong way, but I did find it a little tedious in places."

"Right. Well, thanks for being honest."

Unlike a tennis score, a book can be read subjectively. Why is it that one person loved this novel enough to have a line from it tattooed on her collarbone, but for Judith it was simply "tedious"? And also, couldn't she have lied or just not said she read it?

All evening I'm paranoid and touchy. I must have PMS. I believe that I'm being put on with weaker players as some kind of punishment, or because no one realizes how truly awesome I am. I should be playing with three strong men always. In my heart, perhaps I am a strong, athletic man, and that's why I feel this way. Or maybe I'm just a baby. Judith puts me on with a terrible player against a guy who says he's injured but who whacks the ball as hard as anyone, and then they all want to stay on for another game but I want to get to where the real action is, playing with Del and the better players on Court 5. I have a good set with an attractive woman of about my age named Karen against Debbie and another woman where we win 6–2. But then Del comes to play with me against Karen and Debbie and I'm not sure what's going on because Del seems to be deliberately letting them win. Karen hits the ball hard at him. They flirt. It's all very confusing. Somehow, Karen and Debbie beat us 6–2. Del keeps talking about what good players they are; how they should play together more often. He comments on my bright orange tennis top. It's another thing I've bought from Simona Halep's French Open collection. "Thanks," I tell him, in a *back-off* kind of voice.

I'm not playing well at all. I'm tired, it's getting dark, my blood sugar is plummeting. I miss a couple of easy volleys and flounce off back to the baseline. Del misses most things. I've seen him play against First Team men before and he is brutal. What the fuck is going on here? Eventually I notice that it's 9:00 p.m., that we've been playing an hour longer than I thought. I say I've got to go home and leave them to sweep the courts. As I leave, Del comments yet again about how bright I look in my orange tennis top. I do my best not to snarl back. Afterward I feel ashamed. I am going to have to learn to control my sulks and temper tantrums or I'm not going to allow myself to come back.

I get home to find a well-spoken man named Rex on the phone. He says he's calling about Seniors' Wimbledon. I imagine he's about to throw me out, but all he wants is for me to play in my correct age category, over-40, rather than in the over-35. In fact, I signed up for both. I signed up for everything I was eligible for. I feel as if I have committed something of an offense but it isn't bad enough to be thrown out. In fact, he says he's going to accept me—me!—

although of course I haven't done anything special apart from have the guts to enter something that looked so closed. Later I find out that "closed" in this context simply means that it is a national rather than an international tournament. So it's closed to overseas players.

•

On Tuesday, I tell everyone about Seniors' Wimbledon. Josh is beyond excited.

"Oh my God," he says. "At last, I am actually coaching someone who's going to play at Wimbledon!"

Dan gets all misty-eyed and begins a long, tear-jerking monologue about how far I've come and how I can't ever have thought, when I first came to the Indoor Tennis Centre, that I'd end up playing in a Grade 1. Both Dan and Josh offer to come and support me.

The only person who isn't impressed is Margaret.

"You should do it too," I say to her, knowing how much she loves Wimbledon, how obsessed she is with everything about it. "I mean, you love going to watch tennis there, why not play? It's literally thirty-eight quid. You get to go in the actual changing rooms and everything."

"That's not the point, though, is it?" she says.

"What do you mean?"

"It's a Grade 1. It's not for players like us. It's for nationally ranked players."

"Yes, well, I'm sure if enough of them sign up I'll get thrown out," I say.

But everyone else I tell is very excited, and no one listens when I say that all I did was press a button, that they could enter too if they really wanted to.

•

Tuesday evening I'm back in Canterbury for my first ladies' match for Polo. I'm playing with Alison Meakin and our opponents are Knoll B, from Orpington. I hit with Alison to warm up and she complains that she won't know what to do if there's no pace on the ball. It's the usual rant about dibbly-dobblers.

The poor old Knoll B team is a bit cobbled together. They don't exactly whack the ball that hard, but Alison and I cope fine. We beat the first pair 6–0, 6–0. It's my first proper double bagel in ladies' doubles and I feel a little bad about it. When we shake hands over the net I say to Sylvia, the better of their two players and who was obviously having a bad day, that the score-line doesn't reflect the actual match, and that they didn't play that badly.

"I am disgusted with myself" is all she says.

The next pair go down 6–0 as well. At the next changeover they say things like, "Well, of course, we don't really play tennis, usually. We were just roped in." That, combined with my sudden obsessive need for Alison and me not to drop a game, gets them the next two. Then we close it out to win the second set 6–2.

Apart from the fact that I have not had my serve for the whole evening I've played well. I've sent some lovely little topspin rollers down the line behind the net player on the forehand side. In fact, I think I might like the deuce side again. Anyway, afterward I am happy. I've made an impression, perhaps. I help the stand-in captain fill in the result form. I drive her home. She can't believe I'm forty-two, or that I've only really been playing seriously for a year. I wonder whether anyone will complain that I was too good, and whether Lucille would have dropped those two games.

•

I'm doing Pilates twice a week now, and I'm thinking of increasing it to three times. I'm playing tennis almost every day. On Wednesday I'm feeling tired and achy and tearful, I almost certainly do have PMS, but I play well with Dan that afternoon. Then I have a coffee with David Flusfeder and discover that his book launch clashes with Nottingham. I've also recently found out that it clashes with the graduation ceremonies of two of my favorite PhD students. I should withdraw, but I don't.

I text Graydon in the evening to see if he's on for tomorrow.

Can you do the morning? he texts back. *I know you said afternoon, but I want to go kayaking.*

I tell him I have Pilates in the morning. I explain that I have matches Saturday and Sunday and a tournament the following week, but what about Friday afternoon? No, he's playing Josh in the morning and won't want to play again in the afternoon.

Next week, then, he texts. I am disappointed. Now I have no tennis for Thursday or Friday. But on Thursday morning it's raining and I guess kayaking is off because he texts me first thing to say he can play in the afternoon.

When I arrive at the leisure center just before three, Dolly is on reception, looking oddly glamorous.

"He's already gone down, already paid. You don't have to do anything," she says.

"Your hair looks nice," I say.

She fluffs it up a bit. "I washed it this morning. Anyway, that man, what's his name?"

"Graydon."

"Yeah, Graydon. He's really excited about playing with you. He said so."

"Really?"

"Yeah, and when I said the booking was for two hours he said 'Even better' with this kind of, well, *look* on his face. I think you've made an impression there."

"Wow. Hope I don't disappoint him."

"You won't."

•

The tennis center is full of French kids sitting in circles gossiping. Some of them are playing a sort of tennis in jeans and sneakers. Graydon is talking on his phone to someone about an audition. We go over to Court 4. Jack Law is just leaving.

"Do you know him?" Graydon asks.

"Yeah, from the odd daytime session," I say. "Do you go to those?"

Graydon makes a face. "I used to," he says.

"But you're too good now, right?"

I'd like to say that's it's only Graydon who brags for the next five minutes, but I am guilty too. I say how I used to play Lee but my winning easily each time was probably getting embarrassing for him. Graydon talks about playing with Josh. Says again that he takes a couple of games off him now and then. Aces him. I brag a bit about beating Paul Gregory in the box leagues.

"You beat a man?" says Graydon.

"I'll beat you if you like," I say. But this is not what happens.

We start hitting. I'm nervous, as I always am playing someone new who I suspect might be better than me. My grip is all over the place. I launch a couple of two-handed backhands skyward. A few nice forehands, though, and a couple of good volleys. Then the backhand again.

"Haven't you got one of those nice hard backhands?" he says. "Hasn't Josh taught you that yet?"

"Oh, he has," I say, laughing. "But it still falls apart under any kind of pressure. I'm still transitioning from the one-hander."

We play a bit more. I hit a better backhand.

"Good! That's better," shouts Graydon. I hope this doesn't go on.

I'm really keen to experiment with playing from the baseline, rather than behind it, so I move in, looking to drive volley anything that's long and wondering if I'm capable of half-volleys or doing anything at all with low balls that land at my feet. I dig a couple out and feel quite good about the resulting shots. A drive volley or two.

"Why are you standing there?" asks Graydon.

I laugh. "Oh, just pretending to be Eugenie Bouchard," I say. "Even though I don't really like her that much. Just trying to be a bit more attacking, you know?"

"Sorry?" he calls. "Can't hear you."

We move toward the net. I repeat what I said.

"I can go back to being Rafa if you prefer," I say.

"You do like standing way back behind the baseline," he says. "I talked about it with Josh. And by the time you hit the ball it's so low. It's around your feet."

I sigh. "Yes, well, I hoped I wasn't still doing that."

"You are!" He demonstrates. "It's like all the way down here when you hit it."

"Right. Well, thus coming to the baseline."

We sit down and have a drink. I ask him how he takes games off

Josh. What's his game plan? "Oh, I just wait for the unforced errors," he says. From Josh? Right.

"The thing I like about hitting with you," Graydon says, "is because the pace is so much slower I have much more time to think about my shots."

We agree to begin playing points. Immediately Graydon's whole style changes. I am standing behind the baseline waiting for his hard-hit crosscourt shots. But instead I get a drop shot, and then another one. Real men don't play drop shots. I have never seen Josh play a drop shot, ever. Real men hit the ball hard and if they want a point they hit it past you. I admit I am angry about drop shots in general. But whatever. Graydon serves pretty big. His second serve is big too. When I do my second serve he just laughs. Which, OK, is sort of fair enough in a way, but also a bit rude.

"So this is the great Scarlett second serve," he says, moving to the service box line to receive the next one.

I still win my service game. Then he wins his. We're 1–2 and I'm serving at the other end. He's a good receiver, that's for sure. I've decided to go back to my harder, flatter serve, but it's not working on him, and feeling embarrassed about my second serve means I just end up having to hit more of them. He attacks my first serve anyway. My second serves come back as drop shots. I get to deuce but then he breaks my serve and wins his to love. We change again.

"Are you going for winners?" he says. "Or are you just trying to get the ball back?"

"I think I'm just playing," I say. Although he's found another button to push.

"Go for your shots," he says.

I'm still trying to be nice, and polite, and jolly, so I laugh.

"Yeah, sometimes I have to lose the first set before I do that," I say.

All this is fair enough in one way, but he's supposed to be the opponent. Opponents are supposed to be quiet. Opponents are supposed to win with dignity if they have to win at all. Opponents are supposed to respect you. I can't imagine trying to give pointers to Sylvia after beating her 6–0 the other night. She was obviously a good player having a bad day. Why would I want to humiliate someone when I have won anyway? And Paul Gregory. I could have told him to hit the ball deeper, to be more precise, but he knows that. If I'd said anything at all to him I would have felt like an utter cunt.

I get one more game when Graydon is clearly too nervous to close out on his serve. Then we're into the second set.

"So this is where you start really playing, right?" he says.

But I don't. I can't. I'm not enjoying this at all. He is a better player than me. He's a better player than Dan. I'd like to be able to beat him, but I'm not good enough yet. He is also desperately competitive. He has worked out my weaknesses and is exploiting them. My second serves are still coming back as drop shots. Then finally he hits one that flops into the net.

"Can you try and hit your second serve a bit longer?" he says. "This is ridiculous."

"Why don't you hit your drop shot longer?"

My next first serve just misses the back line.

"That's better!" says Graydon.

"Sorry?"

"That's a better length."

"That was my first serve," I sigh. "Look, would you rather just hit? I mean I really think that this isn't—"

"Go on," he says. "Have your second serve."

Of course it goes in the net. My poor fragile serve, which breaks down with even a mild compliment, let alone a set of outright in-

288 • SCARLETT THOMAS

sults, is now gone. I double-fault on the next two serves. I want to go home. For the next game I just think *fuck you* and I try to hit the hardest returns I can, but I just end up making my arm hurt. I am lost in the rectangle in which I usually feel so good, so right. Still, it's OK. I don't mind losing to a better player; I just wish there weren't all these mind games. Is he doing it deliberately? He doesn't have to. He'd be beating me without them. Just maybe 6–4 rather than 6–2. Although it looks as if he's going to take the second set 6–0.

On the changeover, I'm not happy. But still he chats.

"Those balls I hit long," he says. "It's because, well, playing you is just so different from playing with Josh. I mean, when the balls are coming with basically nothing on them it means I have to generate all the pace myself. Then I end up overhitting."

Did I just hear that right? I did. But I can't storm off at 5–0 down.

"This is going to be the last game for me," I say.

It's only 4:20, but I can't take any more. I pretend I need something in the office and so I go and stand in there until he's gone.

"What was all that about?" asks Margaret.

"That man is completely insufferable!" I say.

But Margaret seems busy with her admin and so I leave.

Later that evening Graydon sends me a text message.

Did I upset you somehow? You seemed upset. And was I to infer that you didn't want to play again?

I wait a few hours and then text him back: *I guess I was a tiny bit miffed when you said how slow I play, lack of pace on the ball etc. A few too many comments/observations overall for me! But fair enough—you are a better player. I thought we were more evenly matched than we turned out to be. So I just thought you'd want to find someone else. No hard feelings though! I'll look forward to your tennis documentary :-)*

He texts back immediately.

Lol . . . I think it was my scary critical upbringing surfacing . . . so sorry about that. I'm also very thick-skinned in the sporting arena and forget that others might not be so (being an actor doesn't help either . . . constant kick-backs and reminders about how mediocre you are).

Lol, I reply. *I am the total opposite of all that!*

Graydon clearly wants to carry on the conversation. I'm becoming uncomfortable. I mean, surely he knew this was not a date, right? That stuff he said to Dolly—I wasn't supposed to take that seriously. Surely he knows I have a partner? Maybe not. He keeps texting into the evening, stuff about the film and TV industry and how it compares to books. He is making the point that everyone is brutal and we must all be quite thick-skinned by now, and I am saying that everyone in the book world is really quite thin-skinned. It's one of those exchanges where he replies immediately and in depth and I take longer and don't say very much. He's actually a much nicer guy in text than he was playing tennis, but I'm still not interested. Eventually he says, *Let me know if you want to hang out at any time.* When I haven't replied by the next morning, I get a message asking me to leave my half of the booking fee with Josh. When I get around to doing this, Graydon leaves me £3 change for the balls.

•

Saturday is our last Kent league mixed doubles of the season. Dan and I start a bit hesitantly against their first pair, Robert and Annette, but end up beating them 6–3, 6–1. We beat the next pair 6–0, 6–0. Afterward we whack the ball to each other for a bit, waiting for the others to finish. I rip one past Dan.

"Scarlett," he says, in a whiny, put-on voice. "Can you just try to hit it a bit harder? Otherwise I think I might hit one long."

Of course I've told him all about my exchanges with Graydon.

"You're quite good. Have you ever thought about becoming a tennis coach?" I say back, which was what someone said to Dan once during a match.

The other team aren't staying for tea, but we all hang around for a bit, chatting about Cheryl's new house in France and the best strategy for a second serve. Someone's put a moustache on Andy Murray. It's quite realistic: bits of hair that someone found somewhere and stuck to his top lip with a piece of tape. While we drink tea, Adam is cleaning the cupboard and vacuuming the office. Dan takes pictures to prove he's done it. Apparently Adam and Josh have been told off by Margaret for being such slobs. I ask Dan if he's playing in the winter leagues with Hayley. If he is, I'm going to have to find someone else to partner me and start grooming them, but then suddenly Dan is asking Adam if he wants to play in our team. "Who would I be playing with?" Adam asks. "Hayley Palmer," says Dan. "Good partner," says Adam.

On Saturday night I dream of the box leagues match I'm playing against Nicholas Handley the following morning. We have both beaten poor Paul Gregory 6–0, 6–0 and since Fin Murray isn't playing, our match is essentially the final of our box. In my dream I lose 6–0, 6–1. I'm up early with a bit of a hangover, eating primal cereal and drinking tea and forcing down some water with electrolytes. The electrolyte tablets do seem to stave off the lower leg cramps I was getting so badly in May and June. I drive off thinking that at least I can't do worse than I did in my dream. At least I have a chance to do better in real life when the loss is in a dream.

Our match is due to start at 10:00 a.m. We've booked one of the indoor hard courts at Polo Farm because there's a junior tournament taking place on all the outdoor courts. But when I arrive, it seems that the tournament is happening inside as well. Nicholas isn't pleased. Simon Grieve comes over.

"What's going on?" he says. "Apparently the system let you book a court regardless of the tournament?"

"Yeah," I say. "It's for our box leagues match. It's kind of a final."

"Right."

"It took ages to arrange," I say. "But I suppose we can try and reschedule."

"No," says Simon. "If you've booked it, you've booked it. Just let us know when you're finishing up."

Simon gets a couple of kids to help take all the mini-tennis stuff off our court. "Enjoy," he says.

Maybe this'll be the time that Simon notices me? I guess they want the court back quickly, but this is not a quick match. We grind out the first set to 5–5 by, rather bizarrely, losing all our service games. I'm using a game plan again, hitting only to his backhand. He comes into the net a lot, but I lob him, just like I did Paul Gregory. I also play some nice forehands down the line, and my usual crosscourt winner. I manage to win a service game at last and then take the first set 7–5.

In the second set Nicholas seems to wilt a bit, and I take full advantage of this. He still loses his serve but I win mine. I'm hitting the ball hard, grunting loudly, generally making a spectacle of myself. I have no idea what I actually look like, but in my head I'm Sharapova, Kvitová, Halep. I want people to look at me and think *She's so good!* I win the next set 6–1. Simon comes over but doesn't say anything about our match. He just starts replacing all the mini-tennis stuff.

•

Josh is obsessed with tennis. He lives for it. I admire and envy his ability to focus all his energy and talent into this one beautiful and pure thing. Whenever I bump into him around the leisure center—as I often do, because like me, he is always there—he is walking fast with a focused, amused look on his face, as if he's just played the most amazing prank ever. As he walks he plays air-forehands. His knees bend slightly, a bit less than they would if he was playing a real forehand, and he reaches in front of him and *swoosh*. And again: *swoosh*. It's a lovely smooth reaching movement.

In the end, perhaps these imaginary forehands contributed more than anything else to my learning topspin. I explained it to Couze last time I was in Devon, and he was very interested, because he always loved ball games of any sort. I told him how you don't hit the ball with the racquet in the way you'd imagine, like side to side. Instead, the action involves the racquet being held in front of you like an upside-down frying pan and simply moved from right to left, over the top of the ball. You don't begin by looking at one face of the racquet and end looking at the other one. Instead, the racquet remains in the same flat, horizontal plane. The top of the racquet at the beginning of the shot stays the top of the racquet at the end of the shot. You never *hit* the ball exactly, you stroke it: the flat face of the racquet smoothing over the fluff on top of the ball. Josh's air-forehand always looks as if he's standing just slightly too far away from his favorite horse and is reaching up and over its flanks, running his hand over the horse's sleek coat. Or maybe he's dusting a shelf just above shoulder height but is again standing a little too far away, like something from a dream.

If you were to look closely at Josh doing this, you'd also see his right wrist as it falls down clockwise, loose and seemingly benign as he comes into the shot, then flicking powerfully counterclockwise as he rises up through it. His fingers are splayed to represent the tennis racquet and the whole thing moves in slow motion, wave-like, through the air. If he did it full speed it would look more like a violent slap, but instead it looks beautiful and serene, like the tide coming in, and in, and in.

•

If I were cool I would travel the country with one perfect tennis dress and a spare pair of knickers and I'd just wash everything in my hotel room each evening, no doubt like people used to in the good old days. But everyone knows you can never dry anything in an English hotel room. Also, I do have what I think is a perfect tennis dress but it's new, and the problem with new clothes is that they might turn out simply not to work, to rub in the wrong place, to make me look fat.

I am trying to transition to white tennis clothes before Walmer, where white is mandatory, and Seniors' Wimbledon, where I guess it will be too. But I feel odd in all white. I feel fat in all white. So I have lots of white tennis outfits that I have never worn and then one backup non-white outfit and also my new US Open Stella McCartney dress, which is a beautiful kind of gold-brown-nude. At home I would drive to a match in just my tennis skirt, but they are very short. In a taxi I definitely need to wear leggings underneath. In case the swimming pool hotel does not have dead bodies, I have taken my swimming stuff. My laptop, to write my book, even though I also have my iPad. Chargers. Ordinary clothes including stuff for if it's hot and stuff for if it's not hot. Two pairs of shoes. Seven pairs of socks. Then there's all the food. There won't be gluten-free bread in the hotel, so I have a loaf of that. Bananas. Apples. Peanut butter in squeeze packs. Crackers. Wraps. I could survive in the wilderness for a couple of weeks on what I have in my bag.

The hotel is really nice. It has a large air-conditioned gym, a swimming pool with no dead bodies in it, a sauna, a steam room, and a nice Jacuzzi. There's one young guy with a couple of tattoos using the gym, then the spa stuff. He tells me how to make the Jacuzzi work properly, and how to get the steam room warmed up. The hotel staff couldn't be nicer. My room isn't massive, but it has a little step up to the door which I can use to do my eccentric calf stretches that, along with the electrolytes, seem to be the only thing preventing my awful, debilitating cramping.

All for £50 a night. The only slight problem is that I have arrived just at the beginning of a heat wave, which I love, but more so in my large Victorian house by the seaside. The sun shines into my hotel room all day. I hardly need the sauna.

Nottingham feels like a city of sport. And I belong! I do! My taxi takes me past Trent Bridge on the way to Nottingham Tennis Centre and I feel a new affinity with professional cricketers—sportsmen of all types. For some reason the affinity is with the men rather than the women. I don't know why.

Nottingham Tennis Centre is impressive. It has a number of indoor and outdoor courts, including its own grass Centre Court with tiered green seating, where locals recently watched Nick Kyrgios beat someone less famous than Rafael Nadal, whom he then beat at Wimbledon. When I arrive there's a national wheelchair tennis tournament taking place on the outdoor hard courts. It's all very professional and snazzy. I find the organizer of my tournament, Peter Whitehead, and pay the remaining £1 of my entry fee because for some reason I was only charged £24 at reception.

But there are several snags. Because there's no official consolation draw, there will be no rankings points for consolation matches. But worse, my over-40 final with Lynn will also only be a ratings match because you need to have more than five people in a draw for ranking points. My dreams are dashed. I should have gone to David's launch like a true friend. This is my punishment. I go to the café and drink peppermint tea because they have no soya milk. I have not had any real caffeine since this morning. My first match is going to be at 2:30. I'm nervous, but excited.

At 1:30, I go to the locker room. I've never spent much time in locker rooms before, but it turns out that these are perfect places for stretching, talking on the phone, listening to music, being naked. They have free toilets. Showers. And a lot of privacy, since girls hardly use locker rooms. After I'm changed, I stretch and dance around, listening to Chiddy Bang. *You can do this*, I tell myself. *You must* do this. *Since you have betrayed one friend, two PhD students, and at least one colleague in order to be here, you'd better win.*

But as soon as I see my opponent, Sumitra, known locally as Sam or Sammie, and described by Peter earlier as "sort of Asian or summat," it is clear that I won't win. She has the body I am working toward. Indeed, she has been through that body and come out the other side. She is pure sleek lean muscle. Her legs look like something you'd find on a thoroughbred racehorse, except tiny. She is skinny, cool, exciting-looking. She is wearing Nike, with the same Asics shoes I wear. Today she is rocking them in grape. Tomorrow she will be rocking them in orange. She is, I hardly need to remind myself, a 5.2. I have never seen anyone like her in Kent, where all the county players look like they could double as rugby forwards or tea ladies.

Peter puts us on Centre Court. The sun is shining. It's such a beautiful setting. There is only one spectator in the stands though:

he is with Sammie. Could he be her coach? Her partner? He's a lot older than her, but then of course my partner is a lot older than me. But he's not here. I'm on my own. I wish someone could see me playing here. It's so lovely.

Sammie is left-handed, which is a bugger, given that I am now programmed to keep hitting the ball to the backhand corner of a right-hander. This throws me, but it wouldn't have been any different if she'd been right-handed. She thrashes me. I do take a couple of her service games to deuce, and win four of mine, but it makes no difference. It's like playing Vanessa Brill all over again, except Sammie is a lot nicer. Of course, she's also a lot older. I think she's closer to thirty-five than forty, but even so. I didn't know it was possible to be like that at our age. Her body! Her forehand! I want everything Sammie has so, so much.

Toward the end of the match I become aware that there is another spectator in the stands. He has a big camera and a tripod and he's taking pictures of us. At least, I assume it's both of us. Suddenly, here on Centre Court, I am not alone. I imagine the flash of one camera bulb and then two—not that you'd even need a flash because of the strength of the sun—and then dozens. I can hear thousands of rapt spectators gasp and sigh and now roar with delight as I play one, then two blistering topspin forehands crosscourt to Sammie's backhand, saving a match point and pushing the score backward from advantage to deuce, and then forward to my advantage. I get the game, but it's not enough. The final score is 6–2, 6–2.

Just before we shake hands at the net, Sammie presses a button on her sports watch.

"One hour forty-eight minutes," she says. "One thousand and fifty calories."

Oh, well, at least I kept her playing for a while. Does playing tennis really burn that many calories, though? It can't possibly. If it did I'd look like Sammie, and I definitely don't.

The photographer is here from Nike, apparently. Sammie—wait for it—*models* for Nike. Dear God. She is everything I ever dreamed of—or didn't know was possible to dream of. Her partner is named John. I guess he's in his early sixties. While the photographer gets Sammie to pose back on the court, John tells me that the match was much closer than the score-line suggests, which is kind and, I suppose, almost true. When she's finished being photographed, Sammie asks me if I want a hit the next morning on the grass courts. Sounds good, I say. We exchange numbers.

Back at the hotel I get in the sauna and then have a swim. I see myself in the gym mirrors on the way out. I look like a wet, fat woman who is literally washed up. Over my dinner of chicken madras with vegetables and a large glass of red wine, I read the Andre Agassi book I've brought with me. It's got to be the greatest tennis memoir ever written. The first scene is the best piece of sports writing I've ever encountered and ends with Andre Agassi and Marcos Baghdatis, having played the most difficult match imaginable, lying almost dead on adjacent massage tables in the locker room, holding hands.

After dinner it's too hot to sleep, and it's noisy outside with drunken guys coming out of a club, so I lie on the bed naked and drink water and read more until finally, at about 3:00 a.m., the curtains start to move in the faint breeze and I realize that at last outside it is silent.

Sammie picks me up the next morning at 11:30 in a very flash Land Rover. She is wearing Stella McCartney for Adidas. Not from this season, some much cooler season from another galaxy. The top is pink with STELLA MCCARTNEY FOR ADIDAS written on it in nonchalant italics. The shorts are yellow. She looks amazing. Why is she wearing Adidas when she's some kind of brand ambassador for Nike? It's uncertain.

When we get to the NTC, Alexandra Valokova is just finishing off what looks like a whitewash against Edwina Jackson. The final set is 6–0. The first was 6–1. Peter says a little grumpily that Sammie and I can't hit on the grass courts now because there are too many matches going on. When I follow him into his office, he starts grumbling about Sammie and "people like that" demanding too much. What does he mean? Is he being racist? Something else? Sammie does kind of swan around like she owns the place, but why not? I mean, just look at her! Then Peter suddenly says that I could have a consolation draw match with Edwina now if she'll agree to it, so I chase her on her way into the café. She's thrilled to have another match, especially as I suggest it might be on Centre Court again.

I feel a bit like one of the eagles circling overhead, my prey in sight. It is extremely hot. Edwina looks a bit knackered. Surely, *surely* this means I'll have a chance against her? All I want is a win, dear universe. Just one little teeny-tiny win. We are not assigned Centre Court in the end, but instead Court 3, which is round the back of Centre Court tucked away in a forgettable corner in front of some loud and dusty roadworks. It's pretty grim, but never mind.

I win the toss and decide to serve. I imagine that Edwina won't be so silly as to put me at the sunny end, since she'll have to serve there next. Just to make sure, I say something along those lines. She shrugs. "I think I'd like to start at the other end anyway." The stupid cow has just put me to serve in the sun! But I am the stupid one really. I should have chosen the non-sunny end and let her choose to either serve in it herself or give me the serve. But whatever, it's too late now.

I feel like I should beat Edwina the way Alexandra just did, with crisp clean winners sparkling through the heat. And I do, more or less, until I am 4–1 up. But then we get into a few long, timid rallies that aren't much better than the ones I used to play. We are fighting over deuces when I should be hammering her into the ground. The sun is much hotter now, and there is no cloud cover. Edwina is one of those players who loses track of the score easily, but then reacts badly when she finds out what it is, rolling her eyes as if I just decided quite randomly that it would be 40–love, rather than winning three points in a row completely fairly. This has begun putting me off to the extent that I am no longer reaching 40–love easily at all. In fact, I have started wishing this would end.

I lose the next game and it's 4–2. Not a disaster, but I need to close this out.

In the next game she quickly gets to 40–15 on her serve. Blast.

"Forty fifteen," I say, as she moves up to serve on the deuce side for the next point. She steps backward, clearly in a huff.

"Sorry, *what's* the score?" she says, shaking her head as if to remove the unpleasant sound that has just entered it.

"Forty fifteen," I repeat.

"What?" she says, shaking her head again and sighing as if I'd given her a large utility bill for a service she canceled three years ago. But she is in the lead and I don't understand what's wrong with her. I mean, what's not to like about 40–15?

"I'm sorry," I say, "but what exactly do you think the score is? Unless it's game, I mean, I don't even understand—"

A light flickers. "Oh," she says. "*Forty fifteen.*" And then she wins the sodding game.

Behind us the machines whir and churn and dig up bits of road for Nottingham's new tram line. It is loud and dusty and still so very, very hot. I thought this match would be easy but it isn't. I start hating myself. I start tightening. Edwina is winning more points now, but because I am tightening, they are longer points and she is clearly tiring. After one long rally, she goes and stands by the fence for a minute or so. After another, she looks like she might pass out. I am finding these exchanges uncomfortably hot and tiring too, but I don't let her see that. I jump up and down a few times so she is under no illusions about how fit I am, how much more I have left in my tank. After I win the first set 6–3, she retires.

I won! Yay. Also: I hate myself a little bit. But she's an 8.1 and I don't care. I finally have a qualifying win. At last.

I go to the locker room and have a shower. Then I go to the café and eat a baked potato with beans. I drink tea. I eat an apple. I watch a men's match. I watch Lynn Coppell beating Emma Kingzett 6–4, 6–3. Lynn looks like a very strong opponent. Oh, well. I guess I'll just use our game to practice something. Maybe I'll go all-out aggressive this time, since it probably won't matter.

Back in the locker room, I change into my next outfit: whites with a neon pink bra. I'm trying to feel energized for this afternoon, but I feel sort of nothing. I probably shouldn't have come here at all.

And then I go out onto Centre Court and completely thrash Lynn.

I'm not 100 percent sure how I do it. I get eleven games in a row but then it hits me what's happening and I can't close out on my serve at 5–0 in the second. In the end it's 6–0, 6–2. It's a fantasy: the kind of perfect game you play in your head before going to sleep. I slip through the points like a knife through butter. Every time I want to play a perfect shot, I do. Crosscourt winner? Yup. Down the line? OK, then! There's something magical about the whole match. It's pure joy.

It's different: *I'm* different. But how? What did I change? The main thing, I guess, is that I decided to go for my shots, to have fun, treat the game like a practice, and just hit the ball as hard as possible. I particularly attacked Lynn's serve, on the basis that she should win her serve anyway and therefore I only needed to break twice to win the match. *So*, I thought, *why not have fun trying to blast it?*

I also tried to stay in my defensive V the way Josh told me. I'm not sure my attacking V was as well organized, but side-stepping diagonally meant that I got to most of her deeper balls. She whacked a few winners down my backhand side, but my movement around the court meant she was forced to take more risks on the angles and a lot of them went out.

I was inexplicably loose and relaxed. My muscles felt good. I just kept thinking that the match didn't matter and I wasn't going to win it anyway so I might as well have fun. And I did. I enjoyed it more than any other match I have ever played. As soon as I come off—feeling happier than I ever have after a game of tennis, possibly ever—I get a cup of tea and call Rod. Sweat drips down my phone.

"I won," I tell him. "I won!"

"Congratulations," he says, and I can hear the joy and pride in his voice.

"I can't believe it!" I say.

"How did you do it? Were you aggressive?"

"Yes," I say. "I think so. I don't really know how I did it."

Lynn drives me back to my hotel, which is lovely of her. Indeed, everyone here is lovely. I'm suddenly so glad I came. When I get back to the hotel I text everyone. Of course, I've been in constant touch with Josh all day. At one point he even sent me a video of him hitting forehands. *Copy and repeat*, his message said. Is he a little bit conceited sometimes? I don't care. He now congratulates me and says that if I could get one more win against an 8.1, I could ask the LTA to bump me up to a 7.2 before the end of the season. So no pressure for tomorrow, then.

As soon as I've finished dinner, I go to my hotel room and start writing notes and trying to analyze what I've done. How did I win? What can I learn from this match that I could repeat? What could have made a difference? Was it the baked potato? The apple? The cup of tea just before the match? Was it because I wore white? I did my hair differently today: a rare ponytail. When did I last play in a ponytail? Maybe it helped somehow? My pink bra. My stretching session in the gym this morning. Playing another match first, but not a long one. The Destroyer, my beloved Destroyer, the racquet I know and feel is different from all the others, and not just because of the red heart dampener that is its only observable defining feature.

I literally have no fucking idea.

•

Sammie texts me first thing the next morning to see if I want a hit at the tennis club just around the corner from my hotel. It's raining quite steadily. She picks me up, even though it's a two-minute walk, and I'm glad not to get wet. Today she is in a white Mercedes. She is wearing another pair of Asics shoes I have almost bought: today's are pink and blue. All her shoes, I learn, are Asics Speed Gels, like my green ones and my orange ones. I suddenly hate my chaste white shoes, bought because I thought I should have them for the grass season, because they are restrained, girlish.

With her pink and blue shoes Sammie is rocking the tiniest pair of shorts I have ever seen on a woman over fourteen and a pink Nike tank top that looks worn, loved, distressed in that perfect way I remember from when I was fifteen and wanted all my clothes to look like that—in some way, I still do. She is thin, she is beautiful. I have the biggest girl crush on her. And she's so nice.

We start hitting. It's great because we both hit hard, both accurately. One ball lasts forever. It feels like hitting with Josh. Unlike Josh these days, Sammie praises some of my shots and even compliments my ball awareness.

"You always know where it's going!" she says. "I never know where it's going!"

I point out that she did OK the other evening. We practice cross-court on both sides and then Sammie suggests that we each serve a basket of balls to the other, who can practice her return. Sounds cool—but I've never done it before. It's amazing! Waiting to return serve after serve I feel more focused and Zen-like than I ever have on a tennis court. I love this: the poise, the concentration. There is nothing in the world apart from me and the serves coming toward me. Breathe. Hit. Breathe. Hit. I return all her serves hard and unselfconsciously. There are no points here, only serves. But I realize at some point that many of these returns would have been winners.

Afterward we chat. She's so friendly and open and lovely. We talk about upcoming tournaments and who has entered what. I go on a bit about Tunbridge Wells and Seniors' Wimbledon. She's worried about her ranking and rating because she hasn't entered very much in the coming months.

"I'm still recovering," she says, looking down at the dark green acrylic floor.

"Recovering?"

"Yeah. From chemotherapy."

Fuck. How is that possible? I've never seen anyone look fitter or more healthy and strong. Fuck.

•

This afternoon I'm playing Emma Kingzett, whom Lynn beat so easily yesterday. Back at the hotel I have a chicken salad with fries for lunch. I only eat half the fries, but it's too much. As soon as I finish, I know I have eaten the wrong thing. I should have had a baked potato, but the hotel doesn't do them.

When I get to the NTC the rain has cleared and it is hot, very hot, and the cloud cover soon gives way to full sun. On Centre Court Alexandra Valokova and Maia Dunn are wrapping up a close match that Maia eventually takes on a tiebreak. I decide at the last minute to wear my new white Stella McCartney dress rather than my orange and blue skirt and top. My dress exposes a lot more flesh but makes me look more of a badass, I think. And it is grass season, after all. Maia is rocking a white Stella McCartney dress and looks awesome in it. I want to look like that too, although maybe not quite so intense. And I don't want to attract insects. I slather on the sunscreen and hope for the best.

We are on Court 2, which is next to Court 3, which is where I had my disastrous start against Edwina yesterday. The roadworks have now moved on a little bit so they are exactly behind Court 2. The sun is blazing. I win the toss and choose to begin at the non-sunny end. I imagine that Emma will then give me the serve too, but she elects to serve into the sun. *OK*, I think. *Your choice.*

But then she wins her serve. And mine. And her next one. I was worried that she would come out a different player today and she has. But I have the Elbow and I have it bad. I can barely hit a forehand. I can't serve. I keep thinking about how I'm not going to beat her love and love now. Surely the only headline worth having from a game like this is love and love. I keep trying not to think about the

LTA and the possibility of going up to 7.2, which I want so much. Yesterday, on Centre Court, playing Lynn, I felt like a true badass. I came out hitting hard. I convinced her to lose. Everything I did screamed winner. But now I'm wondering if Emma thinks I'm an idiot, with my dress and my grunt. I think I'm so amazing but I can't be because she is suddenly 4–1 up.

This set of tennis is possibly the least enjoyable I have ever played. It is so hot, and I like the heat, but our points are long and I am increasingly worried about heatstroke. I've just read about Andre Agassi vomiting into the courtside flowerpot at some hot tournament in the US and hallucinating through the last few games of his match. I do not want that to happen to me.

Emma plays like I played a few months ago. She plays a bit like Siobhan Clarke, but without the edge. Now I find myself also playing like I played a few months ago. *Hit it!* I say to myself in Dan's voice. It doesn't work. *Hit harder!* I try, which is what Andre Agassi's father always said to him. But I cannot convince myself to loosen up. I stayed an extra night in the hotel for this match. I could have gone home a day early to Rod. Thoughts swirl like puke in a sink. The LTA. Josh. I want to be able to text Josh with another win. But soon, conversations begin in my head about my loss. How I will explain it. *Hit it!* I somehow claw my way back to 4–4, then 5–4. I am dripping with despair. Her serve isn't that good but I have no return this afternoon, so we're back to 5–5. Eventually we end up on a tiebreak that really could go either way. I feel like I am sweating blood when I eventually take it 11–9. If that isn't winning ugly, I don't know what is.

For the first game of the next set, her serve, which I win, I feel happy and calm for the only time in the match. I did it. I won a set. Surely she will now cave in and give me the second one, just like Nicholas did in Canterbury. I can breathe. I can hit forehands. But then she breaks my serve and it's fucking game on again. What am I going to do? I know what I need to do. The problem is how to convince myself to do it. *OK*, I tell myself. *If we stay out here for two hours plus, that means heatstroke.* Do I need to grind a win out of this set? No. I only need to win a championship tiebreak. I don't have an amazing record with those, although I won the last one I played. And I won the tiebreak in the first set here, which gives me tiebreak momentum.

So here's what I am going to do. I am going to play totally recklessly, wildly, with no thoughts of winning. I am going to finish every point as fast as I can, win or lose. Even if I give this set away 6–1, I can go for it in the tiebreak. Are you listening, Self 1? *Please* cooperate. Are you in there, deranged monkey brain? This must make sense even to you. I try to unleash myself and quickly hit a couple of balls wide, but then I'm finding the lines and—for fuck's sake, she's getting everything back. These points are almost as long as the other ones were, but I'm winning them. I keep winning them until I am 5–1 up. She serves. I think—*listen up, Self 1, pay attention, monkey*—that I am four points away from a cold shower, a cup of tea, and a phone call to the LTA. Emma hasn't won a service game for a long time, and her only game in this set is a break. But I can't convince myself to hit hard on points this important, so she wins it. So now I am serving for the match. Guess what? I can't do it. It's 5–2 now. In my head I see 5–3, 5–4, 5–5, 5–6, 5–7. *No. I am too hot. Please let this end. Please, please let me win.*

I am not enjoying this match at all.

It's 0–30 after my first two serves. I hate myself. I'm still four points away from a cup of tea. Maybe even more. Maybe I really am going to lose this match. Then Emma's next deep ball falls just on the wrong side of the baseline. I'm almost 100 percent sure of this. As my finger goes up to indicate that it's out, I suddenly doubt myself. Should I be calling it in? I honestly don't know whether it was in or out. It was definitely more out than in and my gut said it was out so I am sticking with out. But if I was up 5–0, would I call it in? Are some of my calls therefore too *kind*? Or am I simply a disgusting cheat? I think she might challenge, but she doesn't.

OK. 15–30. Three points from a cup of tea, cold shower, etc. Earlier, on a key point, I managed my ad-side ace. It was so close to being on the wrong side of the line that I was virtually serving again from the deuce side before she had a chance to call it out. It's my best serve. I try it again now. It nicks the top of the net and lands on the wrong side. Second serve. Out. 15–40. On my serve. At 5–2. She wins the game.

I am sweating badly now. My towel is on my chair, but if there is another changeover it will mean she's taken it to 5–4, which will mean I have to kill myself. I have to win with what I've got. An almost see-through dress, no liquid chalk on my hands, despair, gloom, desperation. She gets to 40–15 again. How the fuck is she doing this? Because she is the one now loose and going for her shots. I am floundering away playing badly from the back while she is playing well at the net. When she comes to the net, I put up easy smashes for her. When I come to the net, she passes me. But I can't lose this set, not now. I know I said I was prepared to do it, but I can't. So I accept that these last points are going to be long. I send her one way, then the other. Get her in her backhand corner and start sending rollers down the line: one she gets back, two she gets back, but the third is so beautifully placed that she can't touch it. 40–30. *Please let me win this point. Please.* She hits a shot wide and it's deuce.

I am two points from the match. Two very long points. I squander three match points before finally sending her off court with a backhand that she hits back for an easy volley into the open court, which I don't miss. I've won. When we shake hands at the net, I tell her that was the hardest match I've ever played. Is that true? I guess I didn't have cramp, which is something. No blisters, no injuries. The heatstroke has not yet begun. Nothing was stopping me winning except myself, and that's why it was so fucking hard. And all credit to Emma—today she was not the player I saw going down to Lynn so easily the day before. She's gracious, but I can tell she hasn't enjoyed this match either.

Afterward, I should feel amazing. I don't. Winning matches is great, but it also feels as if someone has given you a small, fragile bird to carry around all day. If you open your hands too much it will fly away, but close them too much and you will crush it. The bird is beautiful, valuable, but holding on to it is exhausting.

I go off to the locker room and get naked. This time I am not alone, but I find I like the gritty femaleness of the other bodies around me. We are strong sportswomen and we smell of sweat and toil and, in some cases, victory. Then I get the cup of tea I have been promising myself and go to watch Sammie beat Lynn 6–1, 6–1. Sammie misses a lot of shots and comes off saying she has played badly. She is a perfectionist, like me. I know exactly how she feels.

I sit next to Maia, who I'd assumed was some kind of protégé of Sammie's but is in fact a 2.1 who hits with Sammie in her spare time. Is she also some kind of coach? Right now she's filling in a kind of graph—dots in squares, a bit like a cricket scorebook—where she records every shot Sammie plays. And here is something else I realize I want: the nerdy absorption, the utter focus on tennis to the exclusion of all else. How simple life would be if you only loved one thing, and it loved you back. Didn't Heidegger say something like that? Or was it Hegel?

Maia has a wrist support on that looks better than mine. I ask her about it.

"Tendinitis," she says. She clocks my wrist support. "You got it too?"

"Something like that."

"If I can't stop playing and rest it I might be out for a year," she says.

Imagine.

I love tennis. I love competing. I love playing the way I did yesterday. I felt strong, powerful, almost Amazonian. But I am so terrified of matches like the one I had today. I don't want to play like that again, ever. But of course every time there is any kind of pressure on me there is that possibility. I need to learn to relax. Urgently.

After the match, I go for a drink with Sammie and John. He arrives to pick us up in a black open-top 1976 Porsche. When I get in, the car is full of brand-new-with-tags Nike tennis clothes in size XS. In the footwell there is a pile of fresh-looking packets of Wilson natural gut strings. I begin to say that I didn't realize Sammie used Wilson strings but then I realize that these have been bought today, as a result of a conversation I had about strings with Sammie this morning. I start saying that if she wants strings like mine she should get Champion's Choice Hybrid but then I realize that they are rich and they have a stringer who can turn a racquet around in a day, so it probably doesn't matter that the natural gut strings break more easily.

Sammie is sweaty from her match, so we go to my hotel bar, which is anonymous and unglamorous. We get a table in the window. John asks what I want to drink. I can't decide. I need something but I don't want to drink too much. I ask for a gin and tonic but forget to ask him to make it a single.

"So, you're an 8.2," John says to me when he gets back. "You had fun being an 8.2, didn't you, Sam?"

"Yes," she agrees. "That was one of the most fun ratings." She sighs. "Less pressure than now."

"She's on her way to 1.1," says John.

"How do you do it, though?" I ask. "Like, you're really good at winning matches. I'm stuck on 8.2. How do I get higher?"

"It's all about lateral footwork," says John.

"Right," I say. "My coach says it's all about defensive and attacking Vs."

"Well, her coach says it's all about side to side, not back and forward."

"Scarlett has such good movement!" says Sammie enthusiastically. "And did I say she's a writer? She's writing a book."

"How much coaching do you have?" John asks me.

"Maybe two or three hours a week? I have a hitting partner too."

"I do five sessions with a tennis coach every week," says Sammie.

"The head coach," says John. "Fifty quid an hour. She also has personal training three times a week. And every day in the gym doing footwork, of course."

"Amazing," I say.

I calculate quickly in my head. That's going to be more than £500 a week. Fucking hell. Then again, how far off that am I, really, with my travel and hotels and wrist supports and tennis dresses? Where will it get us in the end? We're all going to get old; we're all going to die. Even Sammie can't stay young and ripped forever. Especially Sammie. What will happen when Nike stops sending her free clothes? And when will that happen? Is this a one-bingo-wing-and-you're-out kind of situation? On the other hand, a part of my mind still yearns to know how I can get Nike to send me free clothes. I'm a bit fat, but sort of healthy?

I really enjoy talking with Sammie and John about tennis, but I'm also happy when they move on to a Thai restaurant and I am left alone to have a large glass of red and a beef madras with chips and a side of seasonal vegetables. I wonder what a real athlete would order from this menu and how far off I am. But I am not a real athlete. Or am I? Is Sammie?

Back in my room I ring Rod and bore him with every moment of my excruciating victory. I am bored with it myself. I should be able to blast a player like Emma 6–0, 6–0. I don't know why it is so important to me to have to completely annihilate the opposition. I'm not sure it even comes down to being super-competitive, because I'm not sure I am. It's more that I want to win without trying. Win quickly, cleanly, and decisively, then get the hell out of there. I want my wins to be pleasurable and easy, not painful and hard.

It's still very hot but there are storms brewing. I need to have my hotel windows open, but tonight there are suddenly insects, lots of them, all gathered in a troublingly big cloud outside the bathroom window. They start coming in. *Mosquitos*, I think. *Cellulitis*. Soon they are on the walls, on the ceiling, little black dots everywhere. I cover myself in insect repellent and lie there on the bed with my skin and eyes burning, imagining waking up covered in mosquitos sucking my blood. I decide to ask reception if I can change to a mosquito-free room. But are they even mosquitos? I google images of biting and non-biting insects and I am none the wiser. I go on a BBC site that has a list of all insects and spiders in the UK that bite. There's the false widow I've heard so much about, its shiny abdomen decorated like a muted Fabergé egg. I didn't know that ladybugs bite. There is not a picture of my insect.

I switch off the light that is attracting them and lie down. My neck burns from all the insect repellent. There's a party going on over the street. It's loud: music and laughing. *Fuck this.* I sit up again and shop for tennis clothes on the internet until there are literally none I haven't seen, and then read more of my Andre Agassi book. He's having about as much fun playing tennis as I am. But he's earning millions—and of course winning—and I am doing it simply because I love it. I do love it. I do.

But I know that unlike Andre, if I'd been sent to my local tennis center aged nine to play a guy for a $10,000 bet my father had made, I would have lost. There's a part of me that still believes that if you want something hard enough you can achieve it: that if you believe in yourself, you are invincible. Perhaps all it takes is to win a couple of times to believe you're a winner, and then you just carry on winning, because you believe you will.

So much of sport is what we believe. Do I believe in myself? As I throw the ball up to serve, do I believe it will be in? Be an ace? Sports rituals come about because people believe they help—like Nadal's drink bottles, Sharapova's dark stares at her racquet strings, or Steve Smith's strange rituals between balls on the cricket field. Rugby players might be the worst for this: the goal kickers with their desperate chicken dances and awkward hair-grooming. Of course, if you believe something will help, it does: there have been many, many studies on the placebo effect. But the opposite is also true: there's a lesser-known phenomenon known as the "nocebo" effect where cursed people obediently die, misdiagnosed people develop the relevant illness, and if Nadal's bottles aren't exactly where they always are, he will lose the point.

Back when I used to be into video games, I couldn't play anything where you had to go through the game with one life and when you were dead you were out, like in a tennis tournament. High-pressure stuff in arcades where you'd put in your quarter and see how far you could get on it? Totally not for me, not with my nerves. Each GAME OVER meant starting from the beginning again, which I could not bear. I preferred games where you could shore up extra lives. If I had a new Super Mario game, the first thing I'd do was to gather ninety-nine extra lives, the maximum you could have. Only then could I start. But if I lost even one life, I'd get so worried and I'd become obsessed with replacing it, much more so than actually going on with the game.

10

The Walmer Open

I'm on the phone to the LTA at 9:08 on Monday morning. For someone who is afraid of phone calls, this is really something. The nice young guy I speak to tells me that I won't be able to jump up to a 7.2, but he can certainly take me to an 8.1 now, and I could still get 7.2 in the end-of-season ratings run. I worry that one of my wins was a retirement, which the LTA site said wouldn't count in this situation. But I also have my box-leagues win against a 7.2 man, which, although not officially countable (according to the website you must only beat people of your own gender), must mean *something*. I am ready to negotiate on the nitty-gritty of this.

I can hear keyboard clicks in the background as the guy brings up my record.

"Oh," he says. "Right. Well, I can't see any sign of these wins yet."

I assure him that they are real, but very recent and so might not yet be—

"Oh," he says again. "Wait. You actually have three qualifying losses this season?"

Fuck. Of course. Sutton: Rachel MacDonald and Alexandra Groszek. Canterbury: Sarah Philips. All 9.1s. Shit. It was only after all that, when I started working properly with Josh, that I started winning. It seems so long ago now that I was losing. But yes, it was during this summer season and so I am still trailing these losses. So I'm not going up to an 8.1 now, and if I want to go up in the end-of-season ratings run I will need two more qualifying wins. I am an idiot for ringing up the LTA like this. I feel really, really stupid.

I go upstairs and settle down to the final edits on my novel. I put in a famous tennis player character and some more meditation scenes, which feel like the only things I can write about at the moment. The tennis player in my book is having a meltdown because he can't win any more, and my hippie-wellness character, who should be satirical but is instead just perfect, tells him to simply breathe. If he breathes, then everything will be OK. Can I still do that?

My next session with Josh is hot and intense. We've moved on to two-hour slots now, and he seems to enjoy pushing me to exhaustion. He feeds me ball after ball that I hit down the line, and then I have to do another basket crosscourt before I'm allowed a break. We're training for Walmer but also, crucially, for Wimbledon. I'm sweating so much that I've started worrying about losing minerals and cramping again like I used to, so I now bring about three liters of water to every session. It is all the pale pink color of that stuff you rinse your mouth out with at the dentist, because of the electrolyte tablets I put in. When did I last go to the dentist? Who needs that normal life crap?

"Are you excited for Walmer?" Josh asks in one of our breaks.

I shrug. "I don't know. I mean, there's no ranking or ratings in it, so."

"Literally everyone is there. To be honest, it's the highlight of my year," he says. "People call it the East Kent Championships."

It's true. Margaret was moaning about this just the other day.

She, like me, wants all tournaments to be overseen by the LTA, but the LTA won't let Walmer hold official tournaments because they won't relent on their dress code. On this, I think I'm with Walmer. If you have perfectly manicured grass courts, why wouldn't you want the people who play on them to look perfect, all dressed in white?

A daddy longlegs has been bobbing and looping around our table. Josh catches it in his hands. At first I think he's going to put it outside—the doors are open after all—but instead he comes over and puts it in my hair.

"Oh my God," I squeal. "Josh! Get it off me!"

He giggles like crazy. And the weird thing is that I sort of like this. Is it because this is the kind of thing he'd do to Becky Carter? But would he really? Wouldn't he be too scared of her ice-cool sexiness? But me? On the one hand I'm old and past it, etc. But boys don't usually put insects in the hair of the elderly and the unsexy.

"You know there was a black widow living in here all last year?" he says. "I used to feed it and everything."

"No you didn't. What the fuck would you feed a spider?"

"Little flies."

"Don't lie."

Josh has now got the daddy longlegs out of my hair. I think he's going to take it to the doors and release it, but instead he crushes it in his hand and drops it on the floor. Is this more or less cruel than me, later that day, "innocently" telling Dan that Josh put a daddy longlegs in my hair, and Dan understanding that Josh and I are proper friends now, and that I might even like him more, with his powerful forehands and his cold eyes and his childish laugh?

•

A week or so before the Walmer Open, Josh invites me for a hit with him on the grass at Walmer, where he's a member. I'm so nervous all day. Josh is unpredictable. One minute he'll be acting about twenty years older than he is, calmly telling me exactly what's going wrong with my forehand, but the next minute he can morph into a ridiculous schoolboy, telling me that I need to open my legs more (while this is true, it doesn't stop it from sounding dirty the way he says it). At times he makes me feel attractive—he admires the different-colored bits of KT tape I've started wearing to support my wrist—but at other times he just straight-up laughs at me. Then there was the weird time he told me all about trying to get off with one of the receptionists and what he said made it pretty clear he's still a virgin. WTF?

We are meeting straight after my session with Dan. Of course I don't tell Dan where I'm going. He wants to talk timetables—everything's changing now it's the summer holidays—but I tell him I have something urgent to do in town.

"What?" he says.

"Just something," I say as I rush out of the door and upstairs to get changed into my whites. This feels thrilling and secret but also sort of wrong. What if Dan saw me? He'd know exactly where I was going just by what I'm wearing. But I'm safe as I rush out of the leisure center and get in my car.

The elegant wrought iron gates at Walmer Lawn Tennis and Croquet Club open this time—with just a touch of authentic creak—and I feel as if I am in *Brideshead Revisited*. Josh meets me at the gates wearing whites and his usual knowing grin. Is he laughing at me or with me? It remains uncertain. There are an indeterminate number of elderly people sitting on chairs watching the tennis on Courts 1 and 2. Just beyond Court 7, where we go to start hitting up, some more elderly people are playing croquet. Josh is carrying a plate of cupcakes and sandwiches. He seems to sort of offer them in my direction.

"Thanks," I say. "But I don't really eat gluten, so."

He laughs his cruel laugh. "I wasn't offering them to you," he says. "You think I'd give my cakes—that Margaret made especially for me—to *you?*"

And yet again, I feel twelve.

I worry that I'm going to be too nervous to even hit the ball. Regardless of the giggling and the cake thing, Josh is doing this for free, as a—sort of, I hope—friend, and I am determined not to let him down. Is there any way a player of Josh's standard could ever enjoy hitting with someone like me? I know Dan does; our knock-abouts make sense for him too. But for Josh this is just kindness, which is sort of uncharacteristic, and therefore confusing. Still, as we get going, I play well. And I find I really like the grass. I win several genuine points from Josh, a nice backhand crosscourt flick past him at the net and a couple of backhands down the line. In fact, I realize afterward, on grass it's my one-handed backhand that seems to be doing the most damage. It was the same in Nottingham.

•

"I hate to say this," says Josh during our next session, "but I think on grass it's all about your one-handed backhand. Especially given your opponent."

Josh has already texted me a picture of the draw currently pinned up on the Walmer LTCC notice board (but of course not on the internet). I'm playing Sarah Luckhurst, who beat Margaret 6–1, 6–1 in our Aegon match. That was the day when I beat Cathy in the championship tiebreak and my fortunes seemed to begin to turn. Cathy and I were both the highest rated in our teams, which is why we played each other. Does that mean Sarah Luckhurst is not as good? No, it just means she does not play LTA tournaments and so her rating is always "wrong," in the way that Lucille's rating is wrong.

Sarah Luckhurst was born in 1975, three years after me, and is built like a female rugby forward. Josh and I think that my only real chance is to move her around the court a lot, at least Josh does. Still high from my Nottingham successes, I somehow believe I have more than just a faint hope of winning. In fact, I'm not sure why no one has been in touch with the people who do the draw at Walmer to point out that they have inadvertently put together two very strong players in the first round. Anyway, today we work on how to actually move someone around a tennis court. Josh encourages me to drop balls in low. Not drop shots exactly, just balls that will die mid-service court. I was sort of embarrassed when I did this at Nottingham, but actually it's a good tactic on grass and nothing to be ashamed of. Get someone back on the baseline and then see if they can run in to catch a falling ball. At one point a dog runs in from the grass outside—it's so hot we have the emergency fire doors open—and even he can't get to one of these balls before it dies.

I get home, exhausted, still thinking about my first match on Sunday. I'll need to have a rest day before then. I also need to time my gym sessions so I put on the maximum amount of muscle before then but without leaving myself sore and tired. The other thing is my novel. I've been slow with my edits, very slow, but I really need it done this month, ideally before the Walmer Open begins. In my mind August is all about the Walmer Open, then Tunbridge Wells, then the big one: Seniors' Wimbledon. I'd like to be free of the novel by then. But the more I've worked on it over the last couple of weeks, the more I have started loving it again. It has to be right. But it also has to be done soon.

I start some short-grain brown rice cooking for dinner and go upstairs for my shower. One missed call on my phone. From *Gordian*. God. We haven't spoken for a long time; I haven't seen him since Steve's funeral in 2011. My heart immediately feels heavy. Something must have happened. Could it be Ruth? She's like ninety-something now. All the regret and sadness I feel about that whole part of my life curls into a ball somewhere deep inside me and I go to the bathroom and have my shower. I guess if Ruth's dead he'll leave a message or call back.

If Ruth's dead, will I have to go to the funeral? Will I have to face the brother and sister that I have never known? I'm supposed to be thinking about my novel. Supposed to be teasing out the last knotted strands of plot. But now I'm wondering whether my sister is beautiful and how I will ever explain to her how eighteen years went past just like that and I never got in touch with her once. And also how I got that email from Ruth at midnight one Thursday after yoga back in 2009 that told me not to contact my brother and sister until they were ready: for Alexander this would be before university, for Katherine, afterward. But I should try to make myself available more for Gordian, the bright flame that had no oxygen, the potential philosophical and intellectual star who instead ended up as a bloodstock agent who read commercial thrillers for fun. I cried all night. Then sent her an email reminding her that the main reason I had no relationships with that part of my family was her and her dreadful meddling. She once told me that my stepmother had always hated me. She also made a habit of reminding me that I was not really a part of the Troeller family. Once her "real" grandchildren arrived, interest in me waned. I pointed all this out in my email. I wasn't that nice about it.

If she is dead, of course, it's too late to send a card saying sorry. I'm not sorry, but I would like us to make peace before she dies. *Too late, too late*, says the water in the shower.

I go downstairs, fluff the rice with a fork. The phone rings. It's my mother.

"It's Gordian," she says. "He's got lung cancer."

Fuck.

Oh fuck.

I ring Gordian. As always when we speak, it's as if we last spoke two days before, not two years ago. He's scared and sad. He's going into Guy's Hospital to have part of his right lung removed. I say I'll come and see him. Ask him if there's anything he needs, anything at all I can do. His voice shakes as he tells me he's trying to give up smoking, and how very hard it is, and how his wife has said she will actually leave him if he doesn't give up this time. I suggest a macrobiotic diet and some exercise. He says he can't exercise because he literally can't breathe. I don't really believe him. Anyone can exercise, and exercise cures everything.

•

In my next session with Josh, the Friday before Walmer begins, we work on my serve. I have a real breakthrough.

"You know the way you bend your knees first and then throw the ball up in the air?" says Josh. "Well, that's a completely redundant movement. You do a little bob—like this—and then, whoop, the ball goes up and then you hit it, sort of plop, like this, but if you bend your knees *after* throwing the ball up, then . . ."

He demonstrates. And yes, I can instantly see that springing up into the *strike*, rather than the toss, makes so much sense. I realize that my serve is still more or less the one I had when I was twelve, which I probably developed by imperfectly copying famous tennis players and people in the local park. For a while I added Dan's tomahawk idea, where you sort of "throw" the racquet and use it to slice across the ball, but I prefer a flat first serve. Anyway, now I try bending my knees after I've thrown the ball. Instantly my serve—which was pretty quick anyway, even when it was totally wrong—is about twice as fast. It feels amazing. I do it again. And again. And again.

"Well, there's your first serve," says Josh. I do a few more.

"If you can hit the back curtain after just one bounce," Josh says, "that's what we count as a really fast serve."

I'm a foot or so off. I keep going. Some children who have been playing outside come and stand at the open fire doors to watch. Three little boys and a girl.

"See if you can hit one of the children," Josh says.

The kids seem to love having balls aimed at them, and giggle and run around fetching any that stray out beyond the fire doors, but of course I don't have the power to actually hit one of them.

"Right," says Josh. "Now I'll have a go."

I am amazed when he steps up to serve and the children arrange themselves in a line like little plastic ducks at a fairground. I'm just as surprised when Josh unleashes a full first serve at them. It bounces off the service court line and then hits the girl. For a terrible moment I think she might cry, but she simply squeals and shrieks with pleasure and does a couple of little pirouettes before resuming her plastic duck position.

"Again, again!" they say, and from this moment onward whenever I want to do a wide serve out on the ad side I will tell myself, "Hit the children." No one ever said sports psychology was pretty.

I serve and serve and then we go back to ground strokes. But suddenly something is wrong: My sacroiliac joint, which caused me all that trouble last summer but which has been fine for so long. I really don't like the way it's feeling, not at all.

•

That evening Rod and I go and stay with friends in London. I've been difficult about this arrangement. I've demanded gluten-free bread and non-dairy milk. Now I moan that the bed will probably make my back worse, with only *two days* before the Walmer Open. We don't drink that much alcohol but it's still somehow too much. I eat stuff that is not in my nutrition plan. I completely flip out when one of our hosts suggests that Andy Murray isn't really that good. What exactly is everyone's problem? A person gets to be in the top ten in the world for something. The *top fucking ten*. In the actual entire world. Out of seven billion people this person is in the top ten and yet any idiot at a North London dinner party can dismiss him as "not that good" because he is not number 1.

•

Back home, and it's the night before the Walmer Open. I've DVR'ed a couple of documentaries that are on because of the Commonwealth Games. One is about the Kenyan 800-meter runner David Rudisha's relationship with Brother Colm O'Connell, his Irish coach. The other looks more lowbrow, but still fun: Dan Hoy goes around trying to find out what makes people successful at sport. The Rudisha documentary has not recorded properly and I spend a long time trying to work out how to download it instead, but in the end we get both programs and sit down with a bottle of red to

324 • SCARLETT THOMAS

watch them. Should I be drinking this much before the Walmer Open? Well, my first match isn't until 2:00 p.m., and drinking a bit the night before didn't hurt in Nottingham. And it worked for John McEnroe, don't forget. And Andre Agassi had his wild crystal meth years, not that he won much during those.

Then Rod and I end up having the worst row we've had for over a year. I'm feeling fragile. I still don't know how to cope with Gordian's illness. We're speaking more often on the phone but I don't know how I feel about that. Why does it always have to be when something is wrong? He says he's depressed and wants to die and I really don't know what to say back. Today is also the anniversary of Dreamer's death, and I feel so sad about that. I'm tense and nervous about tomorrow.

The row begins with some misunderstanding about the documentaries. For some reason I feel as if the Rudisha one, the more serious and interesting film, somehow "belongs" to Rod, and the other one "belongs" to me. So when Rod says that something in the Dan Hoy film was boring and almost made him fall asleep, I react as if I made the sodding documentary myself, to which he reacts badly. It is one of those drunken rows I have come to hate so much because now I can't even really say what it was about. Me crying, feeling alone, so alone, while Rod cleans his teeth upstairs. Screaming at him for some reason that he doesn't know me, not at all—which is the opposite of the truth—and that today is a really, really bad time to be having such a stupid row about nothing. I cry for half the night.

•

The next morning I feel just awful. I'm playing Sarah Luckhurst at 2:00 p.m. I eat eggs on gluten-free toast and have a bowl of hot brown rice with honey but hardly taste any of it. I feel sad, in shock, hungover. My back hurts. I have run three packets of contraceptive pills together to avoid having my period during a tennis tournament, but my body has rebelled and given me a period now anyway. I can't remember the last time I felt physically worse than this.

Josh has suggested getting to Walmer early and hanging around to get the feel of the place, maybe hit up a bit, watch Adam, who is on at noon. I still feel a bit sick, pushing open the wrought iron gates, dressed in my best whites. It's another hot day. Rod's playing cricket, but I wish he was here to watch me. I wish we hadn't had that row. Josh is over on the other side of the beautiful lush green courts. He waves and gestures to me to go over and sit with him. I pick up a plastic chair and carry it around past the croquet lawn.

Of course, Josh is not on his own. As I will discover over the course of the Walmer Open, during this week—his "favorite" of the year, remember—he has a permanent entourage. There's his mum, dad, and brother. Two girls he introduces as his god-cousins. An aunt or two. Some of Becky Carter's family. A couple of his friends. The young guys have all been at someone's twenty-first the night before and are battling hangovers. Josh isn't playing until five or six but everyone is here supporting Adam on Court 7 and Josh's brother Bobby on Court 8.

"What we do," Josh explains to me, "is make a big line like this behind the court where one of our friends is playing and basically intimidate the opponent."

Indeed. And here I am, a forty-two-year-old woman dressed in her very best Adidas tennis whites, sitting beside her twenty-one-year-old coach while his mother—presumably not that much older than me—offers to go home and make rice salads for him and his brother. I don't know what to do or say. The god-cousins are fifteen or sixteen. I can't talk to them. But I can't talk to the older people either. I am Josh's friend. Am I Josh's friend? I feel a little like something slightly undesirable that Josh has brought home from school, like something he left in his locker a bit too long. At some point I mention that I've already had six ibuprofen because of my hangover and my back, but this doesn't make me sound at all cool; I just sound old and damaged.

It turns out that Sarah Luckhurst is a friend of Josh's family. Shortly after arriving, she comes and sits next to one of the aunts. Josh nudges me; raises an eyebrow. Here is the person he's been training me to beat. She seems nice. Big and jolly with a kind open face. But I try not to make eye contact.

Adam's match has finished. I go over to the control room—a posh man in a wooden hut—and suggest that Sarah and I begin early and play on Court 7. That way the line of intimidation won't have to move. I realize that some of the line will in fact be rooting for Sarah, but that actually excites me. Josh will be supporting me, right? Perhaps his friends too. Sarah agrees to the early start and goes to get changed. I go and get the match balls and go on court and begin stretching. And from there I can see Josh and his friends and family packing up their picnic rugs and chairs and moving behind some other court, where one of Josh's other friends must be playing. Will even Josh stay to watch me? No. He does call out a *good luck*, though, before he hurries off. I feel like a loser already.

Still, when we start warming up I hit the ball hard, with loads of topspin, just like Teele Annus did at Canterbury. I want to intimidate Sarah, to show her that I am going to be the boss of this tennis match. But my back really hurts. And I have stomach cramps. The ibuprofen is making me feel a bit dull and my head is full of cotton wool. I win the toss and put Sarah in to serve. The first ball is an ace.

Before I know where I am, she is 3–0 up. She has some friends and family watching her. I now have no one. Josh does occasionally drift along to watch me, which is very sweet of him, but I feel like I am letting him down.

"You have to hit the ball harder," he says through the green chain-link fence at the back of the court. "You're letting her dominate you."

The problem is that I have thought so much about the little drop shots and the side-to-side flicks that I have forgotten that my basic game has to be about hitting the ball deep and hard. Instead I hit these pathetic little mid-court shots that she just comes and kills with her lovely forehand. I really want a forehand like that. Better than that. But I'd like to have it for a while on the way up. I mean, I *am* going up, right?

My back hurts. It feels as if the only thing I have is my fragile new serve. I manage a couple of aces, a couple of unreturnables. She has five games and I have—suddenly—three. Am I doing this? Am I coming back, turning it around, dominating her? No. She has the first set, 6–3. And the next one, in something of a blur, 6–1. All I remember is one of her supporters throwing a water bottle over the fence to her. My back killing me. That forehand. Afterward she offers to buy me a drink. It's customary here. But I just want to go home and cry. I say no and realize I've made a horrible faux pas, but I don't care.

I go home and cry and shower and change. Do I feel a little better? When I get back to Walmer I bump straight into Del, from Canterbury. He's there with Stuart and Lloyd and they're looking for a fourth person to have a hit around. Am I interested? Of course. I rush home and change again. Rod suggests that I might be too tired to play another game today, but I need the hard-hitting blur of playing with men. I need someone to whack the ball at me, hard, for the analgesic rightness of me hitting it hard back, with nothing much at stake. We alternate partners, and of all the combinations, Stuart and I do best. When I get home I find he's sent me a long DM on Facebook saying how attractive I am and asking me out for a drink. Oh dear.

•

Monday. I have texted Dan and had no reply. Is he still all right for a 5:00 p.m. start for our first mixed doubles match at Walmer? He has talked confusingly about being triple-booked this evening—he has his adult session to teach and something else to do with his new girlfriend Jody's birthday—so I am worried. I arrive at around 4:00 p.m. wearing my best white tennis dress. Josh is hanging around with his brother Bobby and a nice-looking dark-haired guy I recognize from the day before. Was it his twenty-first or someone else's that they all went to? Predictions are made. Dan definitely won't turn up. Dan never turns up. He hasn't replied to me, so what are the chances of him turning up? But then, at 4:53, he does.

"I am seven minutes early!" he declares to the guys, not making eye contact with me. Is this going to be another one of those occasions when he goes all blokey and ignores me? If so, I am definitely ditching him as my mixed doubles partner. I have Stuart Bennett as backup, although now there's the complication of him asking me out. Why do guys have to make things weird like that?

We start playing just as it begins to rain.

"It's fine!" says Dan.

But then I slip and Sue, the opponent, does too. The match is postponed.

"Can you all play at midday the day after tomorrow?" asks the man in the control room.

We all say we can. Dan finishes coaching his summer-holiday club at midday, but he can probably leave ten minutes early, he says.

The next day I have my first match in the consolation draw. At least at Walmer the consolation draw is taken pretty seriously. Last year Hayley Palmer won it. The prize is a silver plate, which Hayley referred to as the "loser's plate," which seemed a bit harsh. If I am to win the plate I have to burn through three opponents. I can do that, right?

My first match is with a woman named Anna. She's maybe five or ten years older than me, thin, blonde, and a bit ditzy-looking. Rod has come to watch me today, which I am happy about. He sits on a plastic chair just beyond the fence, with that concentrated look he always has when watching sport. After my matches—in fact after any sporting event he sees—Rod knows exactly what actually happened. For me it's often a blur, but he can remember precise scores, dramatic turning points, changes in momentum.

I am determined to stay focused and win this. I get off to a good start, taking the first three games easily, but I have a new anxiety. It's bad enough trying to win against a good opponent, but what about losing a lead against a poor opponent? I just can't bear the idea of it. On the second changeover Anna notices something I've been trying not to acknowledge: a small fledgling bird is kind of dying in the corner beyond the tramlines on the far side of the court. She keeps shooting worried glances at it.

"Is that bird all right?" she says on the next changeover.

"I don't think so," I say. "But I'm not exactly sure what we can do."

I don't like these life-and-death questions. I don't like animals suffering, but do our human attempts to alleviate the pain actually make it worse? Thoughts swirl in my head: my abortion, Dreamer's death, my mum's friend who was killed by well-meaning friends in an ill-fated euthanasia pact. How the fuck am I supposed to win with these dark and heavy thoughts in my head?

Gordian, I think. I'm going to see him soon.

"Maybe your dad could come and help?" Anna suggests.

What? My dad? Oh, right. She means Rod. Is she fucking joking?

"He's my partner," I say. "And no. If it's bothering you, you do something."

She shoots me a look that says I am the most heartless person in the world, puts down her racquet, and then makes a big show of going and moving the bird out onto some leaves. Does the bird even care whether it dies on a tennis court or on some leaves?

I have no idea how I beat her, but eventually, somehow, I do. It isn't pretty. She plays standard local doubles tennis: soft wide serves, long rallies, weird drop shots. She gets everything back. As the match goes on, the only person I hate more than myself is her. My fucking *dad*? What the hell did she think she was playing at? In the end my 7–5, 7–6 victory feels hollow. I go home and drink a bit more than I mean to and have another sad conversation with Gordian. When I tell him about all my tennis, he advises me to take things more easy. "You're no spring chicken, you know," he says. Maybe he's right. I think about when I was fifteen and idolized him so much. I wanted to be in his world of sparkle and glamour all the time.

My next opponent is a sweet young girl named Emily who hits the ball hard but frequently misses the lines she's going for. She's like a kind of proto–Amie Tonkiss. Emily does actually have her dad with her. He's a tennis coach and shouts instructions from the side of the court, which is a little off-putting. I surprise myself by winning this one fairly easily, 6–2, 6–2. Which means, yep, I'm in the actual final—not the actual real one, but the one for the loser's plate.

But before that I have to play my mixed doubles match with Dan.

Does he show up on time? Nope. In fact, he doesn't show up at all.

I've just about had it with him, says Josh in a text message. *Margaret has too. He's just a fucking liability. He came in late this morning and didn't even thank me for setting everything up.*

I am crosser with Dan than I've ever been before. He texts me various excuses: it's Jody's birthday (still?), he can't leave the children alone at the ITC. I know Josh is there too, but Dan says he isn't.

Still, I have a final to play. An actual final. It's supposed to be against Sara Fairclough, but she has a wedding to go to, so at match point in her game against Clare Carter, Becky's sister, she defaults. I'm there to see Sara and Clare's match, and Becky is there too. She's just beaten Sarah Luckhurst and so she's going to be in the actual real final.

"How did you do it?" I say to her.

"You've just got to keep it away from her forehand," says Becky.

Have I just had an actual conversation with Becky Carter?

•

There's no chance of conversation with Becky on finals day. Or with Josh for that matter. As the tournament has gone on I've increasingly felt that if this whole thing were high school, then I am basically the fat friend who lives in Josh's neighborhood with whom he sometimes hangs out in the holidays and at weekends, but would never acknowledge in front of his cool friends.

I'm not even sure why this is, because I am, objectively, sort of cool. I'm a novelist with a diamond nose stud and designer tennis clothes and a love of gin and swearing. But I am old, so old, and not a member of Walmer Tennis Club, and only in line for the plate. Perhaps if I'd beaten Sarah Luckhurst Josh would like me more.

Becky has turned up with two "comedy" visors for her and Josh to wear in the mixed doubles final. They're lime green plastic on a kind of weird toweling headband. Of course, they both look unbearably good in them. They laugh together as they warm up, doing walking lunges around the back of Courts 1 and 2. Walking lunges? I can't even do a simple squat without my knees seizing up. I can't run without my shins hurting. What the fuck am I doing playing tennis? But as always, nothing is going to stop me.

The ladies' changing rooms are next to the bar. Everything here is made of old wood: the walls, the doors, the benches. The little cubicles don't have locks exactly, just brass latches. Over the years the wood has been polished to a pleasing walnutty shine. You can sort of see into the bar from the changing rooms, which means that anyone in there can see the ladies changing. But no one here would strut about topless listening to Chiddy Bang too loud on big headphones, their boobs bouncing inappropriately, would they? *Fuck it*, I'm thinking as I do exactly that. I may not be able to do a walking lunge right now, but I'm a fucking badass, and I'm going to fucking win my fucking final.

Clare Carter's entire family have come to watch her. They sit in a line under the tree by Court 7. Rod is there rooting for me, and Lee has come too. I've invited Dan, but of course he won't show up. He never does. I win the toss and decide to serve. I win the first game to love, and then the second.

On the 3–0 changeover, Josh walks past.

"How's it going?" he asks.

I tell him the score, expecting that he's going to be proud of me.

"Come on, Clare!" he calls out instead.

"Josh!" I say. Surely he should be happy that I'm winning?

On the 5–0 changeover, Clare starts talking to me. She's a very sweet person, but I'm not really in the mood for hearing about how early she had to start at the bakery this morning, which has made her so tired, and how seriously her whole family takes tennis. Of course, Becky's the favorite because she's so talented and always wins, and Clare feels in her shadow because—

What is this, fucking family therapy? Do I get to share too? Because trust me, you don't want to hear about my family, girlie. How about this? One dad died of heroin and the other two have cancer and it sucks being old and not being able to have your dream anymore. Or even do walking lunges.

I take my drink over to the netting and stand quietly, away from everyone.

I win the first set 6–0. On the next changeover, Clare starts doing cartwheels. Her family smile at how cute she is. I go to get my towel out of my bag.

"Why are you taking this so seriously?" she comes and asks me. WTF?

During the next game, I double-fault. Clare's family claps. Really?

"For fuck's sake," I growl. "You're fucking cheering a fucking double fault?" I shake my head and move across to serve for the next point.

Do they hear me? In the moment I don't care. Later, I try to convince myself that they can't have done. But everything that happens afterward suggests that they did.

But in the meantime, I beat Clare love and one. Yep, she got one game. Turns out the double fault galvanized her, and for the next few points she played a blistering, terrifying tennis that she could have used to win the whole match.

But I do it. I win. I shake hands with her at the net and she scurries off to her family, none of whom will catch my eye.

And then something interesting happens. It becomes cool to lose.

Becky loses her final against a girl with a much bigger forehand. She and Josh lose their mixed final. Josh's men's final is embarrassing to watch. Rod's never seen Josh play before, and so he's stuck around, fascinated to see this prodigy in action. What he actually witnesses is a spoiled child who throws his racquet on the ground every time he loses a point and who actually cries after one excruciating rally. After fluffing a volley on a particularly intense point, Josh comes over to the fence and has to be talked down by his brother Bobby as he kind of pulls at his towel in anguish and stamps—yes, stamps—his little foot. He swears, kicks things, throws his drink across the court.

The line of intimidation does not know where to look.

"Well, it wasn't exactly what I was expecting," says Rod, after Josh loses the match.

"Nope. Me neither," I say.

By the time of the prize-giving ceremony, Josh has regained his cool. The picture printed in the local paper has him standing with Becky and Clare, the three of them looking young and blonde and athletic and beautiful. Around them stand older, uglier people, all clutching shiny silver cups and trophies. I'm there with my silver plate catching the light, looking prouder than perhaps I should. But being a winner isn't all that, really. Josh and Becky both look much more like winners, nonchalantly holding the wine glasses they got for coming second in their singles finals. And Clare? She stands there proudly holding an Evian bottle, and somehow in the photograph it looks like the finest prize of all.

11

Seniors' Wimbledon

I t's less than a week before Seniors' Wimbledon and I am still not meditating every day like I should be. I don't feel very calm. It's been hard to get hold of Josh for some reason. After the Walmer Open he suddenly wasn't available for coaching for about ten days. He declared himself "burned out," went kayaking and fishing, and then when that stopped he told me he couldn't coach me because he was hitting with an under-18 who was 750th in the world and would be "too knackered." So the Carters did hear me, then? Or maybe Josh was just humiliated after his loss in the final.

On Friday night Rod and I go to watch *The Apartment* with David Flusfeder and his wife Sue Swift. I'm exhausted, having spent the morning in Guy's Hospital visiting Gordian, who has just had part of his right lung removed. I've tried to explain what this was like to my friends, but it just comes out like the kind of amusing anecdote I normally tell. I had the first panic attack I've had for a long time in the lift on the way up to the respiratory ward. I couldn't breathe, couldn't feel my heart. When I realized how high up the ward was, I didn't let myself get too close to the windows in case I threw myself out. Gordian looked so small and fragile sitting cross-legged on his hospital bed, but also unmistakably still my cool charismatic dad.

On Saturday morning I'm due to play a mixed doubles league match. Dan texts me halfway through the film. *I'm thinking Plough-mans have sausage rolls and sweets.* Being Dan's official mixed doubles partner means I have to shop for the tennis afternoon tea. But I fail to fully unravel Dan's text even when sober, so randomly buy goats' cheese Camembert and salad. I never eat cheese of any sort but at afternoon tea I do eat some. We've won, of course, but I'm a bit more tired than usual. I go home, drink wine, feel vaguely unsettled all night, and then leave early to play a ladies' doubles at Polo at 10:00 a.m. on Sunday.

It's one of those mornings when I forget how to play tennis or why I even wanted to. There are high winds and some rain. Every-one's depressed. My wrist hurts. We lose. If I can't even win a local doubles match, what on earth am I thinking going to play Wimble-don? Even the word is now making me feel sick. I've stopped telling people I'm playing this week and have started hoping they'll have forgotten.

I'm asked to play another league doubles match that will be just as depressing as this one. It's on Seniors' Wimbledon finals day. "Probably," I say. "I'll let you know."

On Monday morning I am worrying about clothes. I've assumed that Wimbledon means wearing white, although no one has said anything. I have three white tennis outfits that I like. One of them is Simona Halep's main Wimbledon outfit. What if I spilled some-thing down one of them, lost another, and then was left with only one tennis outfit for the entire match? I begin to panic. But I don't really need to buy more white stuff, not this late in the season. In a couple of weeks' time it's going to be all about the US Open outfits. Although what am I, a supposedly serious writer, even doing wor-rying about my clothes? It's what I do when I'm nervous, what I've always done. Every job interview or book launch has always been all about the outfit. But how many outfits do I really need? I'm going to go all the way to Wimbledon and then be beaten and come home again. I need my outfit for about an hour, tops. But what if? What if I do get through? It would take a miracle, but miracles happen, right?

I go to an online tennis shop and fill a virtual basket with skirts and tops, but I don't check out. On another site I order more kinesiology tape, and I do check out. Go back to the other shopping basket, look at it, sigh. Do a bit of writing. In many ways it's a normal morning. I mean to meditate, but I don't. Then I go and play tennis for five hours and somehow fit in a five-hundred-meter sprint on the rowing machine as well. "Tapering nicely then?" comments Josh. I spend the night throwing up.

•

I've booked a room above a pub with a good restaurant on Wimbledon Common. Rod and I check in on Wednesday afternoon. My match is on Thursday at 10:00 a.m. I'm anxious to secure a taxi for the morning.

"Where are you going?" asks the girl behind the bar.

"The Aorangi courts at the All England Club," I say. "I think it's Gate 1."

"Sorry," she says. "Where?"

"The All England Club?"

She looks blank. "What's that?"

"Er, where they play tennis?" Still she frowns.

"Like, you know, Wimbledon," I say.

"Oh, I see." She smiles. "You going to watch some tennis then?"

I have a huge tennis bag with me. "I'm actually playing."
"Oh. Right."

•

Last time I came to Wimbledon—the tennis club—you could barely see the place for people. Now, as Rod and I approach in a taxi down Church Road, the place has a mellow end-of-season feel to it. The seats around Court 2 are covered with plastic, which flaps in the light wind. There's some building work going on. Fluorescent tape.

I've never seen the Aorangi courts before. During Wimbledon fortnight, the fences are covered so you can't see who is practicing there, but now they are all open. And they are beautiful: around twenty perfect grass courts under a cloudless blue sky with just a pinch of autumn in the air. There's a large pavilion, too. I go through a door that says PLAYERS' ENTRANCE and feel impossibly excited. I'm a player! At Wimbledon! I wasn't sure how I'd feel here—I have failed, in the past, to be excited about the Empire State Building and the Sagrada Família along with many other great tourist attractions—but this is something different. I feel, however fleetingly, like I belong. I feel like I am not just being allowed to go backstage, but actually to be part of the production. But I'm still so incredibly nervous.

I'm early; of course I am. I go to sign in—the control room is a bunch of elderly posh men with big hardback notebooks—and am told that my opponent, Sue Depledge, has not arrived yet. I last saw Sue playing Siobhan Clarke at Canterbury. She's the second seed here, but I know she's beatable. Still, I must not allow myself to dream. Not here. Anyway, winning isn't the thing. *Writing* is the thing. I'm a better writer than I am a tennis player (although if a fairy came along and gave me one wish right now, I would probably reverse this) and so I am also here in that capacity.

I've had a piece commissioned by the Guardian's *Weekend* magazine. It's going to be about what it's like playing tennis as an over-40 woman, and specifically what it's like playing Seniors' Wimbledon. It's going to be a curtain-raiser for the tennis book as well as a sort of calling card for my new identity as tennis novelist or sports chick or whatever I end up being. It's like the universe wants this: I've also been asked to pitch a regular column to the editor, so I've suggested a weekly fitness slot. I've been enjoying the gym lately and wondering whether I might get a general fitness instructor qualification rather than a yoga course. I don't really like yoga. It's too slow.

So I'm here as a player, which is impossibly exciting, but it doesn't matter if I lose because I'm also here as a reporter, an anthropologist, a participant observer. I know which one I'd rather be, but I can always fall back on the other.

The changing rooms, "For players and coaches only," are staffed by two attendants in pale blue uniforms. Signs on the doors remind players to make sure they wear "almost entirely" white, to only take Evian and Robinson's Barley Water onto court, and if they must drink Gatorade to pour it into an Evian bottle first. I am overwhelmed by brilliant details.

There are piles of white towels on each bench of the changing rooms. These must not be taken on court: only official Wimbledon towels must be taken on court. The white ones are for the players' private use. This is the Ritz of changing rooms, when before I've only been able to get into the worst B&Bs. At the back of the changing rooms is a massage table "for juniors only" and ice that is labeled NOT FOR HUMAN CONSUMPTION.

A couple of weeks ago I played in Tunbridge Wells. It had OK changing rooms with showers but literally nothing else. I went on the train with Rod. As it was all on grass, it was supposed to be a warm-up for Seniors' Wimbledon, but my first match was canceled because my opponent sprained her ankle, and then it rained so much that my second match was moved to clay. My opponent—a nice, short-haired woman of about my age—had once played for the Netherlands. She'd asked me what pro tennis I used to play. Then she thrashed me love and love and I cried and the rain mixed with my tears and I wondered about giving up this whole stupid thing. Rod sat there in his anorak trying to analyze it all. My serve wasn't bad. I did get to deuce on a couple of games. His eventual conclusion was that I gave it my best, but really? She was completely out of my league.

Here, in the Aorangi players' changing rooms, there are not only the fluffy white towels but three different types of deodorant, hair mousse, hair spray, combs, cleansers. I get the impression that if there was anything you needed—anything at all—the attendants would help you, but in a down-to-earth, motherly sort of way. They sit in a little glass booth, reading magazines and filing their nails. Golden oldies are playing on a transistor radio.

It's only really since Nottingham that I've discovered the joy of the locker room. At school the changing rooms were cold, damp, moldy, and apparently haunted. Anyone in their right mind either avoided going in there in the first place or got out as quickly as possible. I was the kid who never had the right kit, or found that my cheese and cucumber sandwiches had fallen into my shoe. I never had a clean, dry pair of knickers to put on after my shower. But as school PE seemed to consist of standing around shivering, I'm not sure I ever needed the shower or the knickers.

Now, though, I understand that locker rooms are where you

can go to think, plan, stretch, be alone. In his autobiography, Rafael Nadal describes his frenzied pre-match activity, all of which takes place in the locker room: he puts grips on his racquets, has his fingers taped, runs back and forth, jumps up and down, and then takes a cold shower. In contrast, Roger Federer apparently sits quite serenely waiting to be called, maybe checking his perfect socks are the same height on his perfect ankles. I'm not sure what I should do. I have ages and ages. I try to breathe. Meditate. Pray. Stretch. I'm so fucking nervous I could die. It's not really that peaceful in here. The place is filling with women, all over thirty-five, but mainly over sixty. One smiles at me as she finds a small gap on one of the benches, but no one else acknowledges me. I don't know anyone here and I feel like an outsider.

There has been a heavy dew overnight, so play is delayed. A voice announces over a loudspeaker that there will be another inspection at 10:30. I saw in the control room that there are lots of singles matches scheduled this morning. At 10:00 a.m., as well as the women's over-40 quarterfinals—which is what I am playing, because there were not enough entries to have a round of sixteen—there are four women's over-65 matches and four men's over-65 matches. At 11:30 there are four over-75 women's singles and two over-80 women's singles. The delay makes people giggly. A group of women in their seventies are all trying on tennis outfits with GREAT BRITAIN written on them. Everyone else is slowly changing into their whites, waiting for their name to be called. It's thrilling, but so terrifying.

People drift out. The changing rooms grow quiet and I notice all the neat piles of clothes: floral knickers, M&S skirts, sensible cardigans. But when I get outside all I see are athletes, and I wonder if there is some magic in these locker rooms. Is this where you go to shed the uniform of wife, mother, grandmother, trustee, respectable member of the Women's Institute, or—who knows?—the CP, and put on a different uniform: badass, number 1 seed, tennis queen? And is it really too late for me to be able to do that too? Could I be wearing a GB tennis outfit in my seventies? Margaret's voice immediately pipes up in my mind: "No. And get over yourself." While it's here, the voice also reminds me that I shouldn't be in these changing rooms at all. This tournament is not for people like me. But I am here, and I'm writing about it for a national newspaper, so.

Josh sends me a text message wishing me luck and reminding me to hit crosscourt, especially if I am nervous. Dan texts me too. I have all kinds of good luck messages on Facebook. I try to imagine that my supporters are here, that I didn't deliberately put them all off. Is there a small chance that I could I do this? Sue is beatable, tantalizingly beatable. I'm an 8.2 with a good recent run of victories over 8.1s. She's just a 7.2, the next step up from an 8.1. It's not as if I am playing a 4.1 or something. She is in the top ten in the country, yet she is within reach.

I want this so much—to be able to say I got to the semifinals at Wimbledon, to receive the huge amount of ranking points, to get one more ratings win. But mainly I don't want to go down 6–0, 6–0. As I walk to Court 17 with Rod, Sue, and a can of match balls, I'm asking the universe: *Please, not the double bagel.* I'm too nervous to speak, so Rod makes polite conversation with Sue. I have no idea what they're saying. I'm trying to focus on the calm green all around me. The beautifully cut grass. The faint birdsong. The vanishing mist.

I win the toss and put Sue into serve. Unless I've been warming up for hours, I always now do this, not at all because of Brad, but on the basis that I can use my opponent's service game as an extended warm-up. It also puts pressure on: you're supposed to win your service games but often serving first means you are serving cold and nervous. It can be a good way to get an early break. But gosh—I didn't realize just how nervous my opponent was going to be. The first three points are double faults. I'm 0–40 up without having done anything. Somehow this unsettles me so much that I manage to lose the next two points off Sue's very wobbly, nerve-wracked second serves that only just make it over the net. But I go on to win the first game. And the second. And the third. Sue's making a lot of mistakes and I am, albeit in a scrappy kind of way, capitalizing on them.

I do not allow myself to think that this is really happening. I've made that mistake before. Instead, I try to focus as Sue struggles with her serve. She really has the yips but I can't allow myself to feel sorry for her. I do a bit, though, and I'm an idiot, calling a serve in when it was probably just out—and then losing the point. My own game is struggling to find any kind of rhythm. I'm not serving that well either, and my forehand has gone a bit wrong. As usual, I'm not hitting the ball hard enough, not playing aggressively enough. I'm afraid to hit the ball hard in case it goes out; bizarrely—for someone deliberately wearing a neon pink bra under her whites—I am afraid to hit my more flamboyant shots in case someone laughs at me. But who? There's no one here apart from Rod, and I know he'll be willing me to hit the ball harder, as usual. Oh, and two supporters of Sue's, perhaps her husband and son. They're so unobtrusive that I almost don't notice them at all.

I've spent the past few months developing my two-handed backhand, which does not seem to want to appear in this match. So I am hitting my one-hander instead: my oldest and in some ways most dependable shot. My second serve involves a grip change from my first serve and today I am so tight I can't even manage that. As always when I am most nervous, I simply flop a pathetic second serve into the box and then despise myself. Against strong opponents who kill these serves, and when I am losing badly, I tell myself, "Just first serves from now on," but more often than not my body just will not do it and, stuck between the serve I want and the one my unconscious seems to want, I end up double-faulting anyway. Today I tell myself—again and again—to hit hard, go for my shots, don't worry if I lose the first set because there are two more left in which to play more defensively if I have to, but my body simply will not do it. It still wants to block, push, play it safe. Why? It baffles me.

However, it soon becomes clear that Sue is doing such a great job of losing this match that all I really need to do to win is remain alive and on the other side of the net. Is that even true? She does hit a small number of amazing shots, and I manage a few myself, but her serve still isn't working. I hold all my serves, except one. I somehow manage to play all the shots that have worked for me this summer on grass: little crosscourt backhand flicks, sliced backhands down the line, drop shots. This match seems to be more about delicate play than power, and I can feel my unconscious rubbing its hands because this is the game it likes best. Low-risk, low-power tennis. My conscious self still yearns to look like Rafa, but it's never going to happen.

I win the first set 6–2. Breathe. Remind myself that this isn't over. How many times does Sharapova lose her first set only to blast her opponent to oblivion in the next two? Am I going to be blasted into oblivion? Sue does come out fighting and holds her serve in the first game of the second set, but then everything goes exactly the same way as the first and I win it 6–2. Even on match point I'm worried that she's going to fight back: take the game, the set, the next set. It's so terrifying, so exhausting, so—

OMG. I've won. I've actually fucking won! I don't believe it. We shake hands at the net and Sue apologizes for giving me such a poor game, for having lost her serve completely. She looks sad and tired. I come off court unsure what to feel. Did I play better than I thought I was playing? I hope so. I must have done. But it doesn't matter: I've got the win. A convincing win. I go up to the control room to find out when I might be playing tomorrow.

"Gosh, you beat the second seed," says the official with a smile, writing the score down in his hardback notebook. "Bravo!"

I am given a phone number on a scrap of paper that I am to ring this evening to find out when I am next on. This is impossibly old-school-glamorous, but what about the internet? Frowns all round. Oh well, yes, of course, if I really want to, I can also find out on the internet.

I go back to the changing rooms feeling a sense of belonging I have never quite had before. I won! Oh my God. I won. I breathe, taking it all in, deep, deep into myself. The attendants on their lunch break in their booth watching *Countdown*, the machine where they wash the white towels, the place you can fill your water bottle ... I love it all and it loves me back. I just want to stay here, inside this feeling, forever. I take the longest shower I have ever had. I use All England Club shampoo, conditioner, shower gel. I take ages combing out my hair, putting on moisturizer, makeup. I belong here. I am a winner.

Lunch—a sandwich using up the last of the gluten-free bread they could find in the Aorangi Pavilion—is the best I have ever had. I drink the most delicious cup of tea. I ring up the pub we stayed in last night and book us in for tonight. I almost didn't bring an extra tennis kit because I didn't want to tempt fate, but luckily I did. I also put an extra day's parking on the car back home in the train station car park "just in case." Only one day though. I know tomorrow is my last day here. There's no way I could make it to the final. Could I?

I persuade Rod that we should stay at the All England Club as long as possible today: watch some tennis and soak it all up. He doesn't need much persuading; it's fascinating here. After lunch we are just in time to see match point in one of the over-85 men's singles quarterfinals. The man who wins—with a hard-hit, sharply angled forehand—has a pronounced stoop, seems barely able to walk, and has a leather wrist support that could have been manufactured two centuries ago.

I think all of us in the over-35, -40, and -45 age groups must feel incredibly young—indeed, this is the place to come if you are middle-aged but want to feel young—and slightly smug because of our just-about-still-functioning fascia, but also a bit worried about what would happen if we ever had to play one of the super-vets. Their skill is unfathomable. On another court, two over-75 men play an amazing point, full of intelligence and grace but absolutely zero footwork, and we all clap. Next to them is a doubles game featuring a pair who look as if they have come straight from *Dad's Army*, complete with long shorts and stern expressions. One of them calls out a crisp "Me" or "You" each time the ball comes over the net. I'm sitting on a bench next to the top seed in the men's over-45 singles, who has also just won his match.

"He's like my doubles partner," I say to him, laughing, the next time the player calls "You" as a winner flies down the middle of the court behind his partner. The next time he calls "Me" he fails to get the shot back and shouts loudly, "Bloody hell!"

"He should get a code violation for that," I observe.

"Yeah, they should take his bus pass away," comments the over-45 guy with a smile.

I love this so much. I've won. I belong here. I'm here at a tournament that I'm still in. I have not been eliminated. I have not been sent home. This is the best drug I've ever taken. I'm completely, utterly in love—with today, with tennis, with this place.

I have already texted Josh and Dan, so now I do a Facebook status update for everyone else. About two seconds later my mother rings.

"My baby!" she cries. "You won!"

"Hi, Mum."

"I'm so proud of you! Semifinals next!"

"Yes, but seriously, this is it. I'm not going to win tomorrow. I'm just going to go out there and try to enjoy it. Relax, have a laugh, you know?"

There's a long pause. "Well, I'm sorry, but I just don't think that's good enough."

"Mum!"

"Well, you're not going to win with that attitude."

"Well, I'm not going to win with your attitude. Can you not see that I am trying to take the pressure *off* myself so I have *more* chance of winning? Do you know *anything* about sports psychology?"

"All right, all right."

"That's it. You are dismissed as my mother. I'm going to find another one. There's plenty of choice here."

We stay until it begins to rain around 4:00 p.m. I go to the control room for a taxi number and receive another scrap of paper with a scrawled number. I ask an official where I should say I am, and he tells me Gate 1 of the All England Club. But the number doesn't work and so I google "Wimbledon Taxis" on my phone.

"Can I get a taxi from Gate 1 of the All England Club?" I say.

"Of which club?"

"The All England Club." No response. "Where they play tennis?"

"Tennis club? Which road please?"

"Church Road? It's really quite a big tennis club."

This is beginning to baffle me.

•

In the hotel room I lie in bed waiting for my iPad to load the over-40 rankings. I should definitely move into the top ten in Kent now, with this win. The ranking points for a Grade 1 are incredible. The system doesn't care that I went straight into the quarterfinals, it wants to give me the points anyway. In my tennis career so far I have managed to amass around fifty-nine points. But for this I will get around five hundred.

But when I click on my name on the LTA website I find that I am already number 3 in over-40 women in Kent, and number 17 nationally. How? Why do I suddenly have 415 points? Oh. I see. I was given a walkover in Tunbridge Wells, and so I got the points for doing absolutely nothing. But wow. This win today means that I will become number 2 in Kent and end up somewhere in the top ten in the country. Me! I start gabbling about this to Rod, but he's not as impressed as I think he'll be.

"Don't focus on numbers," he says. "Just focus on the game."

•

My semifinal is scheduled for 1:00 p.m. on Friday but we arrive around 11:00 a.m. I want to spend more time at Wimbledon as a winner, because I know my time is running out. In theory my game plan today is to be relaxed, play loose and open, because all the pressure is on my opponent, Chantal Kilov. I met her yesterday in the control room before our first matches. She's a thin, fit-looking woman who plays tennis every day, even Christmas. She's a 6.1. She beat another 6.1 to get here. I am an 8.2 and therefore a total underdog. So the idea is that I will have fun and she will not have fun. I will smile, be irreverent, play my best game, while she tightens, plays it safe, and loses.

Hang on, hang on. I didn't realize this was what I was doing. Have I somehow decided that I am going to win this? FFS, that is so stupid. Because of course if I think I have any chance at all of winning I can say goodbye to being relaxed, loose, etc. Indeed, I can already feel it. I am tense, anxious, snappy. I feel my energy draining away as nerves. This was supposed to be fun! I blame my mother. There are good matches going on all around me. It's semi-finals day, after all. One of the women's over-35 matches is awesome, both players hitting hard, deep, crosscourt shots. Do I play like that? I think I do. I hope I do. Perhaps sometimes in practice? I wonder if my match will be put on Court 1 or 2. I feel like having an audience today. I've brought my best tennis dress, although I do worry that it makes me look a bit fat. And a bright blue bra for underneath.

One of the more elderly competitors has fallen asleep on the junior massage table. The attendants are watching a murder mystery on their portable television. I love it here so much. It has the feel of an old-fashioned British institution, like remote studios at the BBC, or Baker Street Tube station when it's quiet. I change, do my hair, fill my water bottles, and try to do my normal stretching routine, but I'm so nervous I keep forgetting which bits I've done. Everything hurts. My wrist, my lower back, my calves. I don't usually play on anti-inflammatories anymore because they make me feel a little dull, but I pop one today.

Chantal walks in and I try not to catch her eye. I can't take any pre-match chatting. I do approximately ten pees between noon and 1:00 p.m. And then our names are not called. I wonder again if the organizers are waiting for an appropriate court for such an important match. This is a semifinal in one of the lower age categories, after all. But when we are called, at 1:40, we are given a pass code for a gate situated way behind the most remote Aorangi courts. "And then you cross a road, go through another gate . . ." So much for having an audience.

Immediately I feel tearful and cross. This is like Leicester all over again. I've come all this way, spent £200 on a hotel, reached the semifinals of a Grade 1, only to have to play my match in what may as well be another tennis club. The whole point of this was to play at *Wimbledon*. Real Wimbledon. My bad mood persists through the warm-up. Chantal wants her volleys too early; she wants to trade winners rather than have rallies; she wants us to serve at the same time. I've ended up at the sunny end, and when she gives me overheads I simply can't see them. More of my energy drains away with being cross, and by the time we begin I feel like I can't be bothered anymore.

This is a horrible feeling to have on a tennis court. This match is what I have dreamed of, trained for. This is, objectively, one of the high points of my entire year. Maybe even the very highest. But I just feel *meh*. There's no audience, no atmosphere. Rod has to watch from an entire court away, because this court wasn't designed to have spectators. He says later it was like looking down the wrong end of binoculars. The part of me that should be OK about losing is actually desperate to win, but the part of me that actually needs to complete this task knows I am going to lose. I need a sports psychologist, but it's too late.

Still, my right arm feels surprisingly relaxed and I seem able to hit some OK shots. I win the first point of the match with a lovely forehand down the line. I've hit it hard! I win the next point as well. Then Chantal wins the next three points to take it to 40–30. Something in me relaxes, but now in a bad way. I've *almost* won the first game, I think. Almost is good enough in this situation, right? But it's not. It can be, sometimes, when your opponent is going to lose as long as you remain steady. But remaining steady with this opponent means she is going to win. Still, I hold my first service game. But it's the only game I win.

The main problem is that Chantal is good. She's not frighteningly good, just good. She is consistent. She plays every point slightly better than I do, which means she wins most of them. I can see her confidence building as mine begins to slip away. I do everything you're supposed to do. I jump up and down, stay on my toes, keep positive. But I can't make myself do what I need to do to win more points. I'm not hitting the ball hard enough. I'm not taking risks. I'm playing stupidly and cautiously and giving her all the opportunities she needs to win. Why am I doing this? Why, knowing now for sure that I am going to lose, can I just not decide to hit out, be bold, go down in flames?

I manage to draw the last game out to deuce by playing slightly better, but it's too late. We shake hands at the net. I wish her luck in the final. I don't feel like chatting so I leave as quickly as I can, tears beginning to come. I really, really want to hit or smash something. There's a bin. I kick it over and walk on, tears now streaming. Rod catches up with me.

"Hey," he says. "Wait—"

But I want to cry without anyone seeing me. We somehow manage to get out of the complicated gate and across the road and back into the All England Club. There are lots of matches going on but for me the spell is now broken. The changing rooms are not magic anymore. I am an outsider again. I have to take a shower, get changed, go home. Then what? Get drunk? What else is there? But I don't even feel like getting drunk. I've been building up to this all summer and I never thought about what I'd do afterward. I pull my phone out of my bag and find an email from the editor at the *Guardian* saying she's sorry, but they're going to pass on the fitness column idea. I'm gutted. What exactly is the universe trying to do to me here? I plod off to the showers and then stand under the water sobbing, thinking of Nadal after he lost the Wimbledon final to Federer in 2007. But I am nothing like Nadal. I am rubbish. I will soon officially enter the national top ten in my age group, but I feel as if I can barely play the game. I'm stupid, pathetic, a loser. I must now give up tennis, this ridiculous passion. I'm too old, too inexperienced, too prone to psychological collapse. Fuck this. Fuck everything.

As we leave, competitors are still milling about. One man carries an ancient leather racquet bag that could easily have been a prop in *Brideshead*. Another man, well into his seventies, rolls on the floor to ease his back. It's a move I know from yoga. All around are posters advertising the next big seniors' tournament, in Woking. I remember that I have entered this, but not paid. I must now withdraw, surely. I mean to do this on the train home, I really do. But instead I text Josh to tell him about my national ranking. *I guess we'd better start making me look like I deserve it*, I say. And then I press the button to pay for the Woking tournament. Well, one more go won't hurt.

•

It's my first session with Josh after Seniors' Wimbledon. He's excited that I'm now number 8 in the country for over-40 women. He asks about my world ranking. I don't think I have one, I say. All I had was that walkover in the one international seniors' tournament I've played at Tunbridge Wells. But do I have world ranking points? Yeah, maybe a few. He looks me up on his phone. Almost drops it. Laughs.

"You don't know your world ranking?"

I shrug. "No."

He laughs again. "You're 131 in the world for over-40 women. You're in the top 150. Oh my God."

He beams. He's proud.

"Wow. But I've got like one walkover and one loss?"

"It's got two wins, two losses here. The walkover's a win, so . . ."

"Oh. Right." I think. "Oh! Seniors' Wimbledon must have counted."

"Wow."

"Oh my God."

We carry on with our session but something has changed. I'm a world-ranked player. Am I playing like one? I'm still trying to work on my forehand. Taking it earlier, higher, hitting it harder. Some of my shots are amazing and Josh is obviously impressed. But after a flat forehand down the line sails way out, he laughs at me.

"That's a shot from the 131,000th player in the world," he says. Which is probably what I am if you take me out of my age group. Probably not even that.

Then later he does a status update on Facebook.

Congratulations to Scarlett Thomas for going from not having a rank-ing in Kent, to breaking into the top 150 in the world for Over 40s . . . all in the space of 4 months!! 2nd in Kent, 8th in GB and 131 on Earth! One very proud coach.

A few days later I'm checking my stats on the LTA website, taking a screenshot to send to my agent to show him how far I've already got this year. When the page loads I see I'm still number 2 in Kent, but I've gone up to number 6 in the over-40 GB rankings. How is this possible? I literally haven't done anything. Maybe someone died, or had a birthday. Who knows how these things work?

So I'm number 6 in the country, but still an 8.2.

I withdraw from Woking. I find I have no appetite for any more tournaments. Not right now, anyway. Until I know that I can have easier, more pleasurable victories, I decide to simply train like mad in the ITC, diet like crazy, and do the fitness instructor course. But being in the tennis center has become stressful and difficult. I'm that woman who played Wimbledon, who has a world ranking. So why then do I still look like all the other middle-aged losers, fluffing easy shots in league doubles matches? Dan and I are still winning most of our matches, but unless we win them love and love I really, really hate myself.

From late September I'm back at work after my study leave, busy with teaching and supervisions. But I still manage to fit in four or five hours of tennis most days. I'm in the leisure center all the time. Rod has decided that the only way he can get to see me is if he takes up tennis as well. Some days I have a coaching session with Josh, two hours of hitting with Dan and then another two hours of hitting with Rod. My whole life in a rectangle, just like I wanted it to be.

My diet doesn't work, so I change it. People around me are telling me not to lose any more weight, but I haven't fucking lost *any*! I count calories, go macrobiotic, then primal, then vegan, then keto. One day I'm bending down to pick up a tennis ball after a long rally with Dan. The green acrylic floor begins to swim and blur and suddenly everything is spinning and I feel faint. I stagger back to my chair by the net, which seems about a million miles away.

"You all right? You've gone pale," says Dan.

"Don't say that," I tell him, desperately chugging water. "If this is anxiety, it'll make it worse."

He looks concerned. "Don't pass out on me."

"OK, you *have* to stop saying that." I tell him that I'm pretty sure this is a panic attack, that I used to have them a lot, back in the olden days when I smoked and didn't have a killer forehand.

But it can't be that. I'm so fit now, and so successful, and so normal, right? And I have my world ranking and—

b r e a t h e

All of a sudden I'm allergic to the ITC. I feel faint every time I go there. Is it the fluorescent lighting perhaps? Severe dehydration? Those bites I got in the summer—did I get Lyme disease or something? I read dark stories about the tarantella, about people who get bitten by tarantulas having to dance out the poison, after which they are either dead or completely cured. Or maybe mine is more of a *Red Shoes* problem; I did begin my adventure in red shoes, after all. I just never realized that they'd take me to a place where I'd be unable to stop. And it still does take me a few more weeks to stop entirely, by which point I can hardly stand up anymore.

Postscript

It's my fifty-sixth session with clinical psychologist Professor Roger Baker, four years later. We do our sessions on the phone now, although we had our first few meetings in Bournemouth, where he has his private practice. Going there was a bit like traveling to a tennis tournament, although I had no racquets and no sports clothes. Rod had to be with me at all times. I needed to lie down a lot. Everything was bright and overwhelming. I couldn't walk even a hundred yards without feeling like someone might need to call an ambulance.

Roger and I are now doing something that he calls "mopping up." I found him on one of the darker, more desperate days of my nervous breakdown. I'd been to a GP who'd said she was pretty sure I had a heart problem and wanted to refer me to a cardiologist. My inner voice, the one I had still not tamed, the one that used to ruin my tennis matches, didn't need much encouragement to start on my "serious health issues." It was a bit like losing a tennis match all over again: a bad shot leads to a bad thought which leads to a bad shot. Now I'd have a vague palpitation followed by a thought of death followed by another palpitation and so on. These would sometimes last all night. I was exhausted. The more exhausted I got, the more palpitations I had.

It was another form of being unable to stop dancing, like the girl in *The Red Shoes*, whirling around and around on my own thoughts.

On some level I knew I was having an epic panic attack. Once my "dizzy spells" became unavoidable in the tennis center, I started having them in the gym and the car. I had them after Pilates and at the fish shop. I had a big one while out running on my own with no phone. I had one on the Tube coming back from a lunch with my agent. I had one after the photo shoot for my Seniors' Wimbledon piece for *Guardian Weekend*. Eventually I was unable to walk down the street without feeling like I had to hold on to something, like my legs were going to give way at any minute.

The cardiologist said I had ectopic beats. That feeling when your heart basically stops and then does two quick thumps? Completely harmless, but yes, very frightening. Liable to get worse with stress, alcohol, and caffeine. The cardiologist did a treadmill test and found I was fitter than anyone he'd ever treated. A win! This made me feel much better. So I tried to go back to tennis, but the dizzy spells still came. What on earth could be wrong with me? What had the cardiologist missed? On one long night when I couldn't sleep for all the torment, some desperate inner wisdom made me go on Amazon and order Roger's book about panic attacks. It became my bible. Which was why I went to see him.

I have now pretty much made peace with the fact that I was a bit of an idiot in 2014, but I still don't actually know what "happened" to me. Some days I wonder about those insect bites. But I had all the tests. Maybe I had them too late? Officially, though, I didn't have Lyme disease, or low magnesium, or low vitamin D. No one really believed in adrenal fatigue, although if it exists I certainly had it. No one suggested I might be perimenopausal, but when perimenopause did properly hit a few years later, it felt quite similar. In those six hellish months of my nervous breakdown I became the type of person doctors roll their eyes at because I'm there demanding yet another test to explain my anxiety and depression rather than facing up to those things. Basically always an idiot then, which maybe explains why I'm still "mopping up" after so many hours of therapy. Will I never learn? Or maybe this kind of learning can't happen overnight.

Does it matter that I can't put a label on what happened to me? I've learned to resist the simple, stay-in-bed-and-be-careful narrative of "I overdid it," although this is the short version of my story I tell to others: "I played a bit too much tennis and then I had to go and lie down for three months." Even the three months is a simplification: my whole recovery took more than two years. I'd definitely increased my volume of training too fast, but over those last couple of months I also overthought everything to the extent that I completely psychologically crashed. The narrative in my head never matched the reality. I thought I was an undiscovered tennis champion, but really I was just a slightly above-average player. And so I guess I did burn out, like a moth sizzling in the plastic tray of a fluorescent light, because I could not keep away from the brightness and the flames: the promise of glory and glitter all safely contained within a seventy-eight-by-thirty-six-foot rectangle.

With Roger, I have relived and processed the abortion I had in 1989. One painful session involved me reading the story out loud several times until it didn't bother me anymore. I have dealt with issues with my family. I have stopped blaming other people for my life. In March 2019, my beloved stepfather Couze died, and while it was one of the most painful things I have ever gone through, I was able to face it like an adult. I was there when it happened, as he slipped peacefully from this world. I helped my brothers carry the coffin at the funeral.

So what needs mopping up? I'm still uncomfortable driving on motorways. I'm scared of cows. I freak out a lot when a low-flying military jet screams overhead. A test I did early on with Roger showed that I am a mass of phobias. I have no other psychological problems—just lots and lots of phobias. So basically I'm fine? No one's 100 percent normal, right? The most important thing I've learned is that the way to overcome anxiety, pain, and fear is to not be afraid. That what is, is. I've also learned not to google any symptoms, ever. To be positive, rather than negative. To commit to growing and changing, rather than staying still. To accept and welcome the darkness if it wants to be there. But on bad days I'm still a bit scared of exercise. And every so often I say to Roger that I still don't understand why I crashed when I did. I was having so much fun playing tennis. It was my joy, my life.

That peaceful, blissed-out feeling I'd get after playing in a tournament, or even a normal long, hot league match, seemed so dependable, but I never considered that I might be abusing a drug made in my own body. I still get the nice feeling sometimes after a run or a bike ride, but it's much harder to achieve and sometimes leaves me feeling a bit jittery and depressed afterward. Such a shame that I didn't realize what I had back then, and that it was possible to destroy it, whatever "it" actually was. There's so much I still don't understand. I have a friend who is at least four years into a similar extreme fitness journey and nothing bad has happened to her. Why me? Perhaps I'll just never know.

When I tell people about my tennis adventure, and what happened afterward, they always ask if I still play. I did try. Even in the six months of total breakdown I periodically tried to go back to the ITC, or to Sandwich, where I could quietly play with only the parakeets watching. But I never quite got over the anxiety I felt competing and so gradually I stopped. I took up ballet instead, and when that started to feel competitive and intense I went back to running, which I'm bad enough at to not be a danger to myself. I've recently taken up cycling, which I'm good at, which is alarming. Do I miss tennis, though? Hell, yes.

ACKNOWLEDGMENTS

Much love and thanks to Rod, who put up with both the incredible highs and the crushing lows of this strange experiment. Thank you, as always, to my family and friends for their generous love and support. A very special thank-you to Roger Baker for helping me to pick myself back up when all seemed lost. And huge thanks to Jack Shoemaker and Dan Mandel for understanding me and my book.

Thanks to everyone who supports me on Patreon, in particular Jelena, Nilufer Gok, Lisa Degens, May Sharpe, Rob Ellis, Sherlock Bones, Marguerite Croft, Kelly Shorter, Evelina Pecciarini, Jim Cappio, Kathy McLusky, Charlie Phillips, Andrew Leader, and Joe Butler.

Thanks too to all my tennis friends and opponents, and everyone I met while completing this book. I have changed many names in this account, simply to respect people's privacy. I have not, however, changed any names where an official record exists—for example in official LTA matches.

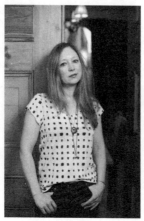

© Ed Thompson

SCARLETT THOMAS was born in London in 1972. She is the author of *Oligarchy*, *The Seed Collectors*, *PopCo*, and *The End of Mr. Y*. The last three books, in addition to other novels, have developed a cult following and sold more than half a million copies worldwide. Her work has been translated into twenty-five languages. Thomas is a professor of creative writing and contemporary fiction at the University of Kent in the U.K.